# The Boater's Medical Companion

CORNELL   BOATERS   LIBRARY

# The Boater's
# Medical Companion

*BY*

ROBERT  S.  GOULD, M.D.

Cornell Maritime Press

*Centreville, Maryland*

Library of Congress Cataloging-in-Publication Data

Gould, Robert S.
    The boater's medical companion  /  by Robert S. Gould.—
    1st ed.
    p.   cm.—(Cornell boaters library)
    ISBN 0-87033-402-6  :
    1. Boats and boating—Accidents and injuries—Handbooks,
manuals, etc. 2. Medical emergencies—Handbooks, manuals, etc. 3.
First aid in illness and injury—Handbooks, manuals, etc. I. Title. II.
Series.
RC88.9.B6G68 1989
616.02'5'0247971—dc20                                        89-43018
                                                                  CIP

Manufactured in the United States of America

First edition

To my wife, Cindy—
my ever-helpful confidante and advisor—
and my three children, Peter, Elizabeth, and John.

# Contents

# Preface

This book is an attempt to bring together in a clear and understandable way methods of dealing with medical problems on the water. The text is not exhaustive in its detail nor complete in its coverage. It is, however, an effort to cover the most common medical emergencies that can occur while participating in boating and water sports. Whenever a variety of treatment choices exist, I have chosen to present the one I would use. When a standard format for treatment is available, such as the American Heart Association's recommendations for CPR, I have chosen to use the standard.

The material covered is presented to assist the mariner and his or her family or guests with understanding and initiating care for medical problems that may occur. It is also meant to assist the reader in performing those tasks necessary to stabilize an injured or ill person until professional help can be reached.

Please note that, for simplicity's sake, from this point on I will use the male gender pronouns he or him as a matter of convention. It should be obvious that she or her may be just as appropriate in most cases.

I have made an effort to cover professional treatment regimens, including the use of prescription medications in some parts of the book. This is to assist the reader when no medical help is available. In no way is this book meant to substitute for proper and timely medical care by competent practitioners of the art. It is my hope, however, that the material contained in these pages will help each mariner feel more comfortable in preparing to leave port for the day.

One of the most difficult parts about writing this book was to convey important information to the lay public who lack the training and experience of a physician. The reader should never forget that the recommendations in this book are a cookbook approach to medical problems and are not designed to confer a doctoral degree. Often the recommendation has been made that the appropriate treatment of a specific problem would be a particular medication. Whenever possible, I have tried to indicate nonprescription medications that are easily available. Substitutions, if available, for prescription medications are included in the list of medications for the cruising sailor at the end of the book. This is in recognition of the fact that most will use this book as an aid to initial treatment prior to bringing the sick or injured party to a doctor. Often, however, prescription medications are more effective or are the only recourse to effective treatment. Under such circumstances, the prescription drug choice is offered. If you foresee the need for such medications, talk with your doctor about your concerns. Bring him a list of the medications that you would like to get and ask for his advice and assistance regarding the purchase of the medications. If he believes that your purpose is legitimate, that you have a reasonable working knowledge as to when to use each medication, and that you are a reliable and intelligent person, he may, quite legitimately, assist you in obtaining small, emergency starter supplies for the medications mentioned. In addition, if you have a specialized medical problem such as asthma, diabetes, or heart disease, he may well have additional recommendations for you. You cannot, however, expect a doctor to write prescriptions for medications for a person that he doesn't know well. An individual may have a condition that contraindicates the use of a specific medication recommended in this book. Your doctor will only know that after a careful assessment of your situation.

Pregnant women and nursing mothers should obtain specific advice from their obstetricians before taking any medication recommended in this book. Some medications have a risk of causing damage to the unborn baby or could be harmful to a nursing infant. You should discuss this with your doctor before using any medication.

My purpose in sharing this complex information is to help you evaluate a medical emergency, determine when medical help is needed, and know how to get that help. You must *clearly understand*, however, that self-treatment of complex medical problems involves some risk. As a physician, I would be giving myself or my family inferior quality medical care if we did not avail ourselves of the diagnostic accuracy of modern X rays, laboratory testing, and the engineering marvels found in a general physician's office. The dictum to physicians to avoid treating themselves is of even greater importance for the general public. None of us can be dispassionate enough to make universally wise decisions about our own medical care. For this reason, it should be clear that the purpose of this book is to give you a resource until proper medical care can be obtained. You can learn to be your own mechanic, plumber, or electrician. The stakes are too high, however, when it comes to your health. You can't afford to make a significant mistake!

# Acknowledgments

When I first decided to write this book, I proceeded with confidence. After all, I have had thirty years of training and experience in medicine. I spent five years in charge of an emergency room on a part-time basis. I have delivered babies; operated in the abdomen, pelvis, and chest; taken care of heart attacks and diabetic coma; and spent two months on a neurosurgical ward. I have set fractures and reduced dislocations. Finally, I have had many years of sailing experience which has taken me over thousands of miles of ocean. For all these reasons, and, because I was willing to undertake the project, Cornell Maritime Press asked me to do so.

After I had finished the first draft and had revised it several times, I began to look over my work critically. I began to have doubts as to its up-to-date accuracy. I realized that, as a urologist, I have a great deal of expertise in my own area of specialization, but that I cannot reasonably be an expert in all fields. Therefore, I asked several of my colleagues, each of whom is currently in active medical practice, to review the work in their specialty and to tell me where I could improve the material.

I am incredibly indebted to the following physicians and one nurse who spent many hours reviewing and discussing the work with me. My thanks go to Joseph Coyle, M.D., general surgery; John Curran, M.D., gastroenterology; John DeLoge, M.D., gynecology and obstetrics; Howard

Kirshenbaum, M.D., cardiology; David Maitland, M.D., general surgery; Clifford Risk, M.D., chest disease; Robin Sendelbach, R.N., cardiopulmonary resuscitation; A. K. Subramanya, M.D., otolaryngology; Harvey Taylor, M.D., orthopedics; Imre Toth, M.D., gastroenterology; and Norman Wald, M.D., ophthalmology.

Additionally, I would like to thank the American Heart Association for permission to reproduce material on cardiopulmonary resuscitation and the Heimlich maneuver; their excellent drawings are reproduced with permission from their *Healthcare Provider's Manual for Basic Life Support.*

The Boater's Medical Companion

# 1. Ground Rules

## TERROR IN THE CANYON

We charged down the big river, our speed increasing by the second as we lurched and bumped over the surging rapids. We clung to our safety ropes and to each other, ducking our heads as the freezing cold water cascaded over our sunbaked bodies. Then the roar started to increase as we swung into the steepest of the declines. It rose to a tumult as six- to eight-foot waves buried our raft. The rubber pontoons arched precariously as we struck the depths of our descent and we were thrown forward against each other. Then, almost as quickly as it arrived, it was past and we drifted downstream laughing and joking with a bravado we did not entirely feel.

The walls of the great canyon rose on either side, brown and ochre, white and yellow; colors of a palette of a master artist, they seemed painted purely for our pleasure. The primeval markings clearly evident in the rocks and the obvious volcanic upheavals of the past lent an other-worldly air to the scene. It was as if we had been transported to another time thousands of years past. I would not have been shocked to see a brontosaurus lift its head in wonder at our passage.

Daylight waned and we sought an anchorage for the night. Dinner was had at sunset and we slept in sleeping bags under the most magnificent sky I'd seen since I last marked constellations in mid-Atlantic.

Dawn came and found me already alert, my senses tingling with the delights of awakening to fresh air and a soft, blue morning sky. The rising sun was just brushing the tops of the distant mountains. The air was cool and the sleeping bag warm and I had no intention of moving for at least another hour. Cindy lay quietly nearby and the kids each had made their own hollows in the soft sand near the river. I started to close my eyes and drift off, snuggling deeper into my sleeping bag.

Suddenly, a piercing scream bounced off the canyon walls. I found myself sitting bolt upright, looking left and then right. The scream was followed by another and another, a woman's voice, and then sobbing and crying and more screams. I leapt out of my sleeping bag and, stopping to bang the bottom of my loafers, I slipped them on and ran toward the sound. Others in our party had beaten me to it. Gail, on holiday with her niece, was holding her foot and crying quietly now.

People made way for me. They knew that I was a doctor. "Looks like she got bit by a scorpion," one of the crew said. "Did anyone see it?" I asked. No one had. I sat down with Gail and held her and rocked back and forth, trying to comfort her. She leaned against me and cried. "It hurts so much," she sobbed. "What was it, Gail? Did you see what it was?" "No," she replied, "I just slipped on my sneakers to go to the bathroom and I felt this awful pain."

We were in a terrible fix. We were five days down the river with no medical facilities nearby, and I had only a very basic medical kit with me. Some scorpion bites are relatively minor, but others can be fatal. Medical wisdom called for a tourniquet and cold applications to the area. The river water was freezing cold. We brought her a pail and put her foot in it. She howled in pain. It seemed to get worse and worse; her foot was starting to swell. Gail was perspiring heavily now and gasping with the pain.

I spoke to Jerry. As our crew chief, he had a small radio transmitter which, if we were lucky, would be able to call in a helicopter medical evacuation. Jerry said he would try to get through. In the meantime I went back to my patient. My mind worked feverishly through the annals and files of my memory for other methods of treatment. Gail was resting against her niece's shoulder, her foot in the cold river water. She kept up a continuous undulating moan. Her lips had a bluish tint to them but she seemed to have no other systemic signs of advancing poisoning. I asked her how she felt. "I can't stand the pain in my foot," she declared almost fiercely. "It seems to keep getting worse." "Cindy, get me a bucket of hot water, fast!" I barked. The fire had been restarted for morning coffee by now as the crew began to prepare breakfast for all the others. "Okay, Gail. Let's switch treatments. This is obviously not helping," I said. "But why hot water? Won't that make it worse?" Gail, incidentally, was also a physician with a practice in radiology in southern California. She couldn't help a lifetime habit of questioning. "It seems to me," I replied, "that I remember learning a long time ago, that a number of spider bites and other toxins are heat sensitive. If I'm right, the heat may inactivate the poison."

We switched her foot to warm water and quickly added hot water to gradually increase the temperature to a level as hot as she could stand it. Within fifteen minutes, the pain had disappeared. The swelling had gone down, and Gail felt like her old self again. Was this a miracle cure? No. I had simply searched my memory for help in handling a problem I had never seen or taken care of before. For Gail, it was fortunate that I could remember. This book has been prepared to help *you* deal with similar difficulties.

## YOUR MEDICAL COMPANION

The world is a wonderful place—until you get sick. Nothing transforms an otherwise happy, confident adult into a confused and frightened innocent more quickly than illness. As difficult and traumatic as an injury can be, the fear it generates can be even more incapacitating than the injury itself. Most illnesses and injuries are simply routine and easy to take care of. Very few, however, feel that way to the patient.

It is my hope that your fears can be assuaged by using knowledge and advice based on years of experience. With full confidence that everything is under control, you will be able to relax under the stress of illness. This relaxation should translate into making clearer decisions, initiating treatment earlier, and focusing on what you can do to heal yourself and others. This is far better than allowing a situation to degenerate into raw panic.

One of the most important things for an injured or ill person to know is that someone is there who can take care of him. Oftentimes a feeling of helplessness overtakes a sick person. The value of having someone sit quietly with him and hold his hand cannot be overestimated. If someone cares, it is healing to the soul. If that person should also have some basic knowledge and confidence in taking care of the patient, the good vibes are almost overwhelming. Under such circumstances a feeling of peace and tranquility will descend over the sick person. This can be tremendously beneficial to his state of mind and aid his speedy recovery.

Just as it is important for the patient to feel that he is being cared for, so also is it helpful for the rest of the crew to know that something is being done. Even the caregiver himself feels better when doing something constructive and healing—so prepare yourself. Each and every one of you can be a healer. Each and every one can and should be able to be relied on in an emergency! Finally, even if you are by yourself, if you have the basic knowledge behind you, if you have prepared, then you will be able to focus on what to do to care for yourself rather than fall apart with fright.

This book is meant to be read. It is not to be used solely as an encyclopedic resource. The principles of treatment outlined are based on common sense and experience. Only a reasonable degree of comfort with those principles will allow you to translate such information into effective action when circumstances demand it.

In years past, it was felt that medical knowledge was too demanding a discipline for more than the most rudimentary understanding to be acquired by the layperson. Today it is recognized that public education and awareness are crucial to the early recognition of medical problems and prompt institution of treatment. This does not require deep and involved study. It does not necessitate an advanced degree. Learning about the human body and how it works is fun. It's interesting. It's about YOU!

Master the principles outlined in this book and you can be confident of managing 98 percent of the problems you are likely to encounter. You may need to get additional professional assistance in many cases, but you can start things off right! Most importantly, you can give yourself and your crew the confidence that the right first aid or initial treatment decision will be made every time.

## GETTING HELP

Circumstances in boating offer challenges to the usual routine of picking up the phone or hopping in the car to drive to the emergency room. You may have powered to your favorite lunch spot down the coast in a protected little lagoon. You may be anchored in a quiet but isolated harbor tucked into a small island with a summer community squirreled away on the other side. You may even be tied up at the dock in a fancy (and expensive) marina within hailing distance of a great city. But in each of these cases, certain daunting problems arise: How do you use the radiotelephone when the skipper is sick? Who do you call? Where is the best place to get help? How do you know if the professional hovering over your mate is competent and skilled? Although each individual circumstance cannot be predicted in advance, several suggestions can be made to improve your chances of getting the right help.

## USING THE RADIOTELEPHONE

In 1971, my wife, Cindy and I, along with our seven-year-old son Peter, decided to participate in a Buzzards Bay regatta. We sailed in the smallest boat in the fleet, a Paceship 23. Lowered clouds and twenty-five-knot, gusty winds reminded us of the northeaster that had passed through the area the previous day. As we shot across the starting line and drove out of protected waters, seas rose to twelve feet. *Little Dove*, our small pocket cruiser, rose to each crest and drove forward with green water pouring over the coaming and into her self-bailing cockpit. We stayed up in the middle of the fleet, footing quite well until we reached a position about four miles from shore. At that point we began to drop back and boats we had easily passed slipped by us.

I was on the helm and asked Peter to look below. He quietly asked if there was supposed to be water in the boat. Securing the tiller, I looked below. Water was filling our boat. The bunk cushions were already floating! I furled the genoa and dove below decks. The only seacock was secure. I spent thirty minutes with a bucket, heaving water into the cockpit while the boat tossed and bucked like a rogue stallion possessed.

I managed to get the water level down to my ankles, and, cold, wet, disoriented, and exhausted, I crawled out into the cockpit to lash my safety harness to a suitable cleat. An enormous wave of nausea rolled over me and I clutched my abdomen with two fists and gritted my teeth. A moment later I cried out, "Cindy, I think I'm going to die!" I could not see that my poor wife had been staring at my staggering and retching bulk with horror. She blurted out in panic, "What do I do? How do I call the Coast Guard?" I threw up over the side and turned back to her weakly to explain that one doesn't call the Coast Guard for seasickness and to ask her to please take me home.

This story points out that many spouses, children, and other crew do not take the opportunity to learn how to use the radiotelephone found on most boats today. Frequently, it is because they are on the boat somewhat reluctantly. It's *his* idea and anything she does to participate is only going to encourage him! Furthermore, all those buttons and dials are very intimidating. Hopefully, this story will point out the very real need to understand how to use your radio to get help.

The VHF radiotelephone is a very simple device (see figure 1). Its range is twenty-five to fifty miles depending on atmospheric conditions, the height of the boat's antenna, and the height of the receiving antenna. It has an on/off switch. This is usually also a volume control knob, just like that on an ordinary portable radio. It also has a squelch knob which is usually the wider part of the two-level volume control knob. The outer part is the squelch and the inner part the volume. The purpose of the squelch is to eliminate static. If the squelch is turned up too high, however, you not only will eliminate static, you'll also eliminate weaker signals. If the squelch is not turned up enough, static will make it hard to hear. I think that it is important to state that radio equipment is being constantly updated electronically. Dials and switches on your radio or mine may, in someone else's boat, be simply push buttons. The principle will still be the same. Once you have learned to use one radio, you will be able to use them all.

The second control knob is the channel selector. Sometimes there are two knobs here, one to control the numbers one through nine, the other to control the numbers ten through eighty. Thus 06 is channel six and 26 is channel twenty-six. That's pretty tough stuff, right?

Other switches may be two- or three-way switches that give you choices. An important one is the channel switch that directs you to 16/Wx/Normal. By directing this switch to 16 and turning the radio on, you will be listening to channel 16, the emergency or calling channel. When you want to listen to a weather forecast, switching to Wx and placing the channel selector to 01, 02, 03, or 04 will give you your local weather. The selector number varies depending on what station(s) you are near. Selecting "Normal" will give you your choice of dial-in channels that will allow you to dial in the previously mentioned number channels. This is done with the rotating control knob(s) mentioned in the previous paragraph. Newer radios may simply have a button for each channel. Sometimes the radio may have a W in place of one of the numbers in the channel selector knobs. This would then be the weather selector switch.

Another two-way switch will say Hi/Lo. You will usually want this on Hi. This is high power output from your

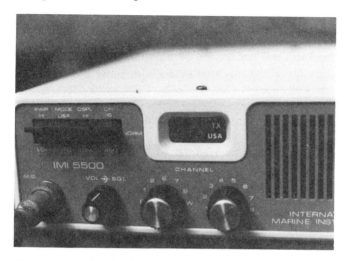

*Fig. 1. Typical radiotelephone controls*

transmitter and should be used at all times unless you are in close harbor contact with your calling party. The final two-way switch will say USA/ITU. Leave this on USA if you are in U.S. waters; ITU is for radiotelephone usage in European countries.

Now let's see how to work this gadget. First, turn on the on/off volume control knob. Set the three-position channel selector switch to 16. This is always the channel that you call out on. Turn the volume control all the way to the right (or on) and the squelch all the way to the right (or off). You will hear a loud sound of static. It should be downright annoying! Turn the volume down until it is simply a little too loud. Then turn the squelch slowly to the left until the static disappears, but no farther. You have just adjusted your radio. It will now perform beautifully.

Pick up the microphone, which is attached to the radio by a flexible, coiled insulated wire. You'll find a button for your thumb on its side. Hold the microphone in your right hand. If you press the button, your radio will transmit a signal, but *will not receive anything*. If you let the button go, the radio will receive others' signals, but *will not send any*. Your radio cannot do both at the same time. When you want to talk, press the button and talk. When you have finished your statement, release the button to hear what the response is.

Your radio has been assigned a radio call sign by the FCC. The owner of the boat should affix this in a conspicuous place near the phone. An example might be WYR 8756. In an emergency, you may dispense with its use, but it should be used whenever possible. It helps to identify your vessel. By convention, the letters are never spoken as letters but as identifying words. B and D sound the same, but Bravo and Delta are clearly different. In the above example, you would identify your boat name and give your radio call sign as "Whiskey, Yankee, Romeo, eight, seven, five, six" (See figure 2 for the complete radiotelephone alphabet). If you learn your call sign now, you won't ever have to think about it again.

In making a call for assistance, you must weigh the urgency of your call. Is it simply for advice? Is it to ask for help, but no one is at risk of life or limb? Is it an outright emergency? If you are simply asking for advice, then call the party you are trying to reach three times, identify your boat's name and call sign, and request that they answer your call. If you wish to place a nonemergency call to the Coast Guard, you would do the following: Turn to channel 16. Listen for 10 seconds or so to make sure that you are not going to interfere with another vessel's call. Press the button on the side of your microphone and keeping it pressed say slowly, in a strong voice, "United States Coast Guard, United States Coast Guard, United States Coast

| **A**lpha | **H**otel | **O**scar | **V**ictor |
| **B**ravo | **I**ndia | **P**apa | **W**hiskey |
| **C**harlie | **J**uliet | **Q**uebec | **X**-ray |
| **D**elta | **K**ilo | **R**omeo | **Y**ankee |
| **E**cho | **L**ima | **S**ierra | **Z**ulu |
| **F**oxtrot | **M**ike | **T**ango | |
| **G**olf | **N**ovember | **U**niform | |

*Fig. 2. The radiotelephone alphabet*

Guard. This is the *Adventure*, the *Adventure* (or whatever the name of your boat is). Please come back." Listen for at least a half minute for a response and then repeat your call. You may have to repeat your call every minute or so for three to five minutes or even longer in order to gain attention. Oftentimes, the radio operator on the other end of the line is tied up with another call on channel 22 or is monitoring other traffic. They are usually quite conscientious and will respond as soon as they can.

If you have a serious injury or medical problem facing you and you need immediate assistance, then precede the above call with the word Mayday. This comes from the French, "m'aider!" which is translated "help me!" The call Mayday is for true emergencies only. All marine traffic hearing such a call will cease transmitting immediately and record everything said by the station calling for help. Assistance may be offered by any vessel if it is determined that it is in a better position to help than anyone else.

An emergency call would announce: Mayday, the name of your vessel, your current position, and the nature of your emergency. To make an emergency call, press the microphone button, hold it, and say loudly and clearly,

"Mayday, Mayday, Mayday. This is the *Adventure*, the *Adventure*, Whiskey, Yankee, Romeo, eight, seven, five, six (your radio call sign here). I am a mile due south of the Buzzards Bay Entrance Tower, and I have a passenger who has had a heart attack. I request immediate assistance. Repeat, I request immediate assistance." Stop transmitting, take your finger off the microphone transmit button, and listen. If you hear no answer in one minute, repeat the message.

One thing should be obvious here. Some preparation should be done in advance of your telephone call. Figure out to the best of your ability just where you are. Are you near some identifiable landmark? Is there a buoy nearby? If there is, go over and identify its number or letter and stay near it. It will help someone find you in a hurry. A few minutes spent at this time will save your rescuers hours of futile searching for your boat. Write down exactly where you are if possible or at least where you were at a specific earlier time and what direction and speed you sailed or motored since. Write down the name of your boat and your radio call sign. Then, you can turn to your radio for help.

You will now get a response in this form: "This is the United States Coast Guard, Point Allerton (or wherever they are calling from) to the vessel calling. Please repeat your message." You will then respond (without the Mayday) by saying, "This is the *Adventure*, the *Adventure*. We are one mile due south of Buzzards Bay Entrance Tower and have a passenger with a heart attack. Can you help us please?" At that point the Coast Guard will advise you to switch to another channel (probably channel 22) for further communications and will advise you how they will offer assistance. You must then switch your three-position channel selector switch to "normal" and dial the number 22 in with your rotating channel selector dials. The number 22 will appear in a lighted window indicating the channel you have selected. When you have changed to this channel, call the Coast Guard again saying, "United States Coast Guard, this is the *Adventure* on channel 22. Do you read me?" (That means, "Can you hear me?"). All further communications will be performed on this channel releasing channel 16 to other potentially urgent calls.

Obviously, it will be a lot less stressful for you to learn how your radio functions before an emergency occurs. So, practice, practice, practice—and have fun. Practicing emergency calls of course, should not be done with the radio turned on. Just practice with it off. Use the radio for legitimate purposes every chance you get.

The following information may also be helpful to you. Each channel designation on your radio has been assigned a specific function. The ones you might most commonly use are shown in italics. Channel 6 is safety. It is for intership communication when safety in navigation is required. Channel *16* is the distress, safety, and calling channel. This is the channel that you use to call another boat or a shore facility to gain their attention prior to switching to another working channel. It is also the channel to use to call the Coast Guard for help. It is the one channel routinely monitored by everyone who has a radio on. Channels 9, *68*, *69*, 71, *72*, and 78 are for noncommercial (that's you) boat-to-boat or boat-to-shore communications (calling marinas). Channel *13* is for navigation and is often used by bridge tenders or by vessels in close quarters wishing to communicate with each other to help prevent a collision. Recreational boaters frequently will call a drawbridge operator on channel 13 to obtain the times available when the bridge can be raised or simply to alert the operator that a boat is on the way. Channel 22 is for the Coast Guard for urgent messages and communications. Channels 24, 25, 26, 27, 28, 84, 85, 86, and 87 are assigned to commercial radiotelephone marine operators. They can connect you, for a fee, to the mainland telephone system. *Eldridge Tide and Pilot Book* lists the commercial radiotelephone channels for the East Coast of the United States. Channels 01, 05, 12, 14, 20, 63, 65, 66, 73, 74, and 77 are reserved for port operations and seldom involve the recreational sailor. Channels 07, 08, 10, 11, 18, 19, 79, 80, and 88 are for commercial vessels only. The U. S. government reserves channels 21, 23, 81, 82, and 83 for its own use. Channel 15 is an "environmental channel." Channel 70, which used to be available for noncommercial operation, is now reserved for "digital selective calling," which involves using a different technology. Since it is used for distress and general-purpose calling for digital selective units, it should not be used by recreational boaters. Weather channels commonly used are W1, W2, W3, and W4, but in some parts of the country, W5, W6, and W7 are also in use. Listen and you will hear which channel your weather is on.

## MEDICAL EVACUATION PROCEDURES

Once a decision has been made to evacuate a member of a ship's crew, a request is made by radiotelephone to the Coast Guard. Several steps must be taken by the vessel and her crew in order to prepare themselves for the evacuation.

The ship's radio must be left on and tuned in to the appropriate channel. The Coast Guard may recommend that you monitor channel 22 or the calling channel (16). Before you disconnect your call, ask them what channel they would prefer you to monitor. If possible, leave a person on the radio to maintain communication with the dispatched vessel. It is preferable that your radio be placed in or near the helm so that you can communicate with your rescuers and still be able to control your vessel. Depending on the circumstances, either a ship or a helicopter will be sent to your aid.

Prepare the patient for transfer. If it is cold out, warm covering to minimize hypothermia is a must. Keep the person comfortable. If possible, put a life preserver on him. A Class I preserver with the increased buoyancy provided would be best. Remember, there will be a time when the person will be somewhere between your boat and the rescue craft. Under the circumstances of a medical evacuation, it is unlikely that he will be able to help himself if he should fall in the water.

Prepare your boat for the evacuation. Remove all loose gear, pillows, and lines from the cockpit. They could trip the rescuers or entangle the rescue craft, probably at the most inopportune time. Accurately pinpoint your vessel's position and, if it varies from the position you gave to the Coast Guard, tell them of the change. To help them find your vessel, they may ask you to talk continuously into your radio. They will then be able to focus in on your radio beam with an automatic VHF direction finder and locate you more quickly. If it is night, activate every light you have aboard so that you can be seen like a Christmas tree. Have flares conveniently available so that you can set one off to bring your rescuers to you more quickly if you can see them, but they don't see you. Finally, head your boat into the wind so that your rescuer can more easily approach your stern.

If you are to be assisted by a helicopter medical evacuation, several very important points must be understood.

First of all, *never touch the cable, basket, or litter which is being dropped from a helicopter until after it has touched the water or the boat!* It will be highly charged with static electricity and can deliver a severe electric shock until it has first been grounded. Second, never attach any line from your boat to the basket, cable, or litter. This could cause the helicopter to crash and could seriously damage your boat and cause fatalities.

If there is inadequate or inexperienced help available in your boat, the helicopter may dispatch a rescue swimmer. He will be a trained emergency medical technician (EMT) and will be able to direct the rescue. The helicopter can then deploy a basket with a cable. When this has touched the vessel or the water nearby to eliminate the static charge, it may be brought aboard. If the person to be transported is ambulatory, he will be able to step over the bar and into the basket. If conditions are calm, the helicopter may be able to hover in position to await this transfer. Never, however, allow the person to get into the basket until a reasonable amount of slack has been placed in the cable attaching the basket to the helicopter. Otherwise, the rise and fall of the boat in a seaway or an unexpected air current could cause the basket to lift suddenly and injure the patient. If conditions are unfavorable and there are winds that are too strong or seas that are too high, then unclip the basket from the helicopter before you put the person inside. The helicopter will rise out of the way and will come back down again with its cable after the person is safely inside. Again, when the cable is slack, attach it by the clip to the basket. The helicopter will gradually lift off to draw the basket out of the boat. Stand by to ensure that it does not become snagged on your boat's lifelines or rigging. The basket is capable of holding up to 600 pounds and usually is used for one adult or, on occasion, two, or for an adult and a child. Three children may be raised in a basket, but the preference is for an adult to accompany a child.

If the person must be raised in a litter as would be the case with a serious back or neck injury, then a litter will be lowered from the helicopter. Again, let it strike the water or the deck of the boat first to eliminate the static charge before touching it. This item will be deployed with a long 350-foot line attached. This line has a weighted end. It must not be attached to the boat, because of the dangers spelled out above. It will be used by the boat's crew to steady the rising litter on its way back to the helicopter. If the steadying line is not used, the litter would start to spin in the wash from the helicopter's rotors. When the litter has reached the copter, you should throw the steadying line overboard.

As these maneuvers are being performed it is critical to prevent the helicopter's cable or the trailing line of the litter from becoming entangled in the boat's rigging or propeller. If available, one of the boat's crew should be assigned to keep watch constantly on the helicopter cable and to assist in keeping it free. If a basket or litter must be brought below to carry out the injured party, always disconnect the hoisting cable first. Upon leaving the boat, the victim should be carefully instructed to keep hands and feet inside the basket or litter during the hoist. This is to help prevent unnecessary injury upon reaching the helicopter.

Helicopter rescues are carried out by trained professionals; However, they involve substantial risk to all involved. They should not be requested unless more conservative measures are not likely to allow the patient to survive.

## A CLASSIC MEDICAL EVACUATION

On a September day in 1988, Carl and Betty (not their real names) left their slip at the Norwalk Yacht Club and set off for a relaxing day sail. It was a Sunday afternoon and they had just had a light lunch. The weather was pleasant and calm with a light breeze brushing the surface of the waters. Betty was a novice sailor. Married for less than a year, the couple enjoyed their cruises together and had joined the Corinthian fleet in their sail to New England waters the previous summer.

Upon setting out for her first sail aboard "Snowshoe," Betty had asked Carl how to use the radiotelephone. "I figured that it might come in handy in an emergency someday." Betty could not have been more right. After an hour or so of sailing, Carl complained that he didn't feel very well. He commented on a pain in his right shoulder and in his back. "I don't feel right . . . I think we ought to go back." Betty was accustomed to handling the tiller, but had not actually commanded the entire boat herself before. Furthermore, she was not trained in coastal navigation and had no idea where they were.

As they slid off downwind, heading back toward the harbor, Carl tried to pull in the mainsheet and stopped, "Honey, I can't do it."

"I'm going below to call for help," she responded. Carl sat down on the cockpit seat, put his head beneath his knees for a few moments, sat up and simply fell over and landed on his side. Betty was a nurse and immediately recognized that he had stopped breathing. His color was terrible. She shook him hard and he started breathing again.

He had a pulse and was breathing but was otherwise unresponsive. Hurrying down below to the radiotelephone, Betty prayed that she would remember how to use the device. Unfortunately, the phone was tucked away in the forward cabin and when she used it she could not see the cockpit or her husband. She turned the radio on. The unit automatically switched to channel 16 and she picked up the microphone, pressed the switch, and called, " Mayday, Mayday, Mayday, my husband has lost consciousness." She proceeded to give them a description of their boat, the fact that they had a mainsail and a jib up and gave the radio audience the number on the mainsail. Then, panicked that she could not see how Carl was doing on the floor of the cockpit, she left the radio to run back to see how he was. Meanwhile, the Coast Guard was urgently calling the vessel in distress to establish where the call was coming from and more details about the problem. In the meantime, Carl had regained consciousness and was struggling to his feet to come below into the cabin. As he reached the cabin floor, he developed crushing chest pain and was forced to lie down on a berth. Betty went back to the radio. The Coast Guard was frantically trying to reach her. They needed a position to effect a rescue. The problem was that she didn't know where they were. She called to Carl for help in pinpointing their location. He was able to relate that they were about four miles southeast of Green's Ledge. Going back to Carl, Betty could see that his color was pale and that he had severe chest pain and shortness of breath. The Coast Guard asked her to go on deck and give them some landmarks. On deck she searched the horizon. She could see the Huntington smokestack and took a bearing on it with the ship's compass. She relayed it to the Coast Guard. Within fifteen minutes, the Darien, Connecticut, police boat pulled up alongside, and a few minutes later, so did the Coast Guard. "Do you have any oxygen aboard?" she asked. The police boat did and brought it aboard. Expertly, the crew of the two rescue boats transferred Carl to a stretcher and over to the Coast Guard boat. One of the Coast Guard crew stayed aboard *Snowshoe*, and Carl and Betty were whisked to Eaton's Coast Guard station where a fire department ambulance complete with EMTs and paramedics was waiting. After stabilizing Carl, starting an IV, and running an EKG, they transferred Carl to the Huntington Hospital where he was able to receive T.P.A., a new clot dissolver. After transfer to a larger institution in New York City, Carl was found to have a single blocked artery to a portion of his heart. This was opened up with a balloon catheter (a procedure called an angioplasty). Carl has since done very well and is recuperating nicely. Good samaritans brought their boat back to Norwalk.

Betty's comment after all this is that, "In spite of being a nurse, I was frightened to death when I was faced with this crisis." The following are her recommendations: First of all, know everything you can about the boat, the way it works, and how to use the radiotelephone. Second, learn something about navigation so that you, as first mate, know where you are at all times. Third, make sure that your radiotelephone is installed in a place where it can be reached from the helm. If it is not in the proper place, have a repeater installed near the helm, so that the phone can be used by one person who doesn't have to leave the wheel or tiller in an emergency. Finally, know everything you can about how to take care of a medical emergency before it happens. Advance planning and training will help anyone to react appropriately when the chips are down. Without this, your reaction times are bound to be slower and the chances are you will do the wrong thing.

## HOW TO PICK A DOCTOR

If you have medical difficulties in your own home waters, you will most likely have previously established sources for medical care. These may be based on relationships with a family doctor or internist, your local hospital, or the requirements of your insurance coverage. In today's market you should verify that you have insurance coverage outside of your area. Many of today's HMO (health maintenance organization) and PPO (preferred provider organization) plans do not provide routine health care outside of their organization or will do so only at some cost to you. True emergencies are usually covered, but you may not want to travel all the way back home to have some routine matter cared for. If so, then plan to pay the bill, unless you have additional coverage with a private health insurance carrier or a broad national agency such as Medicare.

When you are outside of your home waters, how do you find a good physician? There is no absolutely tried and true technique, but the key here is to ask questions. If you need to go to a hospital, ask the local people which is the best hospital in their area and why. Ask the local druggist; he may also be able to recommend a competent family practitioner, internist, or dentist for you.

If you need surgery—and it cannot reasonably be postponed until you can get home—ask the examining physician (probably the local emergency room physician) who is available in the community. Get several names and then ask him who he would choose for himself. Get as much information as you can about this new doctor *before* you see him. Is there a reason that this doctor is being recommended rather than someone else? It may well be that it is a Saturday night and he is the doctor who is on call for that specialty and you are lucky to get him! If you have time, you may wish to get confirmation from someone else in the community (druggist, physician, the nurse in the emergency room, an anesthesiologist). Call your own doctor at home. See if he agrees with the treatment plan. Ask him if he knows someone that he would prefer in that community.

When you meet the physician or surgeon who will be responsible for your care, don't hesitate to ask appropriate questions. Apologize for your concern, but explain that it is difficult for you to start with a new physician in a strange community when you have a serious problem to deal with. Ask him who he is. Is he a specialist in the field who customarily manages such problems? Where was he trained? (Have you ever heard of it?) Is he board certified? Has he had experience in handling cases that are similar to yours? If not, would he recommend someone else who has? Look at him critically. Does he appear confident and capable? Do his hands shake? Is he much too old—or perhaps too young for you to feel comfortable with? Obviously, there are times when speedy help by a professional, *any* professional, is preferable to an unnecessary delay to get just the right one. Like so many other things, judgment is the key to making the right decision.

Once you are comfortable with the doctor you have chosen, then find out what his treatment plan is. Make sure that it has been explained to you in a way that you understand. If you don't like the options given to you, ask what other choices there are. If there are other options, ask about the advantages and disadvantages of each. Why is he recommending one particular option? If there are no other choices given you, and you don't understand or like what you are being told, you may ask for a second opinion—if there is time. If a delay is likely to cost you your life, put your life in his hands unless you totally lack confidence in his thinking or ability. If you are comfortable with the doctor and he offers you a reasonable treatment program, then simply authorize the treatment and get on with your life.

Once you have done your homework, met your doctor, received satisfactory answers to your questions, and understood and approved your treatment plan, then relax.

You are in good hands and a professional will now guide you back to good health.

## PRIORITIES IN AN EMERGENCY AT SEA

When an injury occurs, someone needs to take charge of the boat to order priorities. This is often spoken of in the medical profession as triage. Nowhere is this of greater importance than after an injury at sea. Often, the boat is pounding or plunging over and through waves and the ship's motion will prevent proper care of the injured party. Furthermore, under the stress of an emergency, other crew are at risk of injury too. Several factors must be taken into consideration.

First of all, how big is your crew? With a large crew, each person can be given a different job. With a short-handed crew, one or two persons must do it all and should prioritize the duties depending on the situation. Obviously, it is difficult to plan in advance for every possible crisis, but the following principles apply.

If the boat's motion is extreme, bring the boat into a position where it will ride easier. Trying to remove an injured party from the pitching, slamming foredeck of a boat in a storm at sea is likely to result in further injury to the patient and, perhaps, his rescuer. On a sailboat if there is enough crew (at least two people in addition to the injured party), the boat can be effectively run off before the wind. This will usually ease the motion dramatically. For safety's sake, drop or furl the mainsail first. This will decrease the sail area, slow the boat down, and diminish the risk of an accidental jibe with the further risk of damage to the ship or her crew from a boom that is out of control. Strap the boom down to prevent it from swinging. Turn the boat under jib or genoa control only and head downwind. With the motion thus eased, one person remains on the helm, while a second crew can effect a rescue of the injured party on the foredeck.

If, on the other hand, there are only two of you aboard and one of you is injured, then heave to. This will ease the motion of the boat, allow you to leave the helm untended, and enable you to assist your injured mate with lowered risk. To do this, the most effective method is to furl (or lower) your jib or genoa. Sheet the mainsheet in tightly, and then turn the wheel or tiller to head the boat into the wind. The mainsail alone is unlikely to develop enough power to drive the bow through the eye of the wind and it will head up, lose power, and fall back. If you lash the tiller or tighten the wheel lock in this position, she will continue to head up and fall off, effectively stopping all forward way. If you had a storm jib up in the first place, then you might try to tack through the eye of the wind without releasing the jib sheet. This will effectively place the jib on the wrong side of the wind (aback). If you then, having completed that first tack, turn your wheel or tiller back to head back toward the original tack, the boat, again, will be unable to develop enough drive to power through the eye of the wind and will lie peacefully. Many modern sailboats, however, will not lie comfortably with a backed jib. They do not have a long enough keel for stability with this amount of sail forward and they will lie beam on to the seas causing severe rolling. If this occurs, then try the first technique with the mainsail alone. Once the ship is under control, then the injured party can be approached, transported to a safer and warmer environment, and treated appropriately. Keeping these principles in mind will help prevent further injury.

A powerboat operator should slow his boat to the minimum speed needed to maintain steerage. A slow motion forward, directly into the seas, will serve to diminish pounding and minimize roll. The powerboat operator who is alone at the helm with an injured mate on the foredeck must place his engine in neutral. A sea anchor of adequate size may then be let out from the bow. It will serve to keep the boat's bow into the wind and prevent severe rolling or capsize. The injured party may then be brought to safety.

## MEDICAL TREATMENT PRIORITIES

In the same manner, priorities have to be clearly in mind when you have a crew member who has been seriously injured. The priorities of treatment are in the following order: breathing, heartbeat, bleeding, broken bones. What I mean to say is that it is of the highest importance to ensure that the injured person is breathing or his brain function will cease in a very few minutes. Secondly, and perhaps of almost equal importance, the heart must be pumping to circulate the blood to bring oxygen from the lungs to the brain. Then, when the above have been assured, attention can be given to controlling serious bleeding. Finally, fractures and dislocations can be splinted to prevent further injury. The management of the unconscious victim is discussed under head injuries in chapter 2 and under cardiopulmonary resuscitation (CPR) in chapter 4.

## MAN OVERBOARD PROCEDURES

It is also critical to know what to do if a crew member has gone overboard. Safety at sea mandates that every precaution possible be taken to prevent this critical situation from occurring. Unfortunately, it does occur, and every boat operator should know how to handle such a crisis.

**Sailboat Procedures.** Much of the information learned about such procedures for sailboats is contained in a report by the Safety at Sea Committee of the United States Yacht Racing Union. Some six hundred separate trials were carried out on the water by the U.S. Naval Academy and the Seattle Sailing Foundation. The basic principle to learn is to kill all speed on the boat immediately. Do whatever you must, but stop sailing! Generally, this involves heading up into the wind and going into irons. At the same time, deploy your man-overboard rescue device. Several are available on the market. A Lifesling (a horse-shoe-shaped sling made of flotational material and attached to a 150-foot floating line) or other flotational device with a long line attached to your boat is appropriate. If you have a main and jib up, tack without releasing your jib sheet, and begin to circle the victim. With the wheel hard over, the boat will begin to run off downwind and then jibe as you continue your circle. The person in the water should be able to pick up the long line. If you have a full crew, drop the jib after the first tack, and continue the circle under mainsail alone. Then start your engine (keeping it in neutral) and drop or furl all sail. This technique helps prevent the boat from getting too far away from the person in the water. If the boat moves forward at six or seven knots, you can be too far away to see the person in the water in just a few seconds. If you have the extra crew, assign one person to do nothing else but keep an eye on the person in the water and to constantly point at him so that others can see where he is. Under spinnaker, head up at once as above, but just before tacking, ease the spinnaker pole forward toward the head stay and drop the spinnaker on deck inside the pole. The tack is then accomplished under mainsail alone.

Rescue can then be attempted by the most reliable method available to you. If the person in the water is uninjured, he may be able to assist in the rescue. Position the boat about one-half boat length downwind of the person in the water and throw a flotation device with a line attached for him to grab. He can then be hauled in. A "throwsock" type of heaving line can be thrown into the wind. By placing the boat downwind of the person, you ensure that the boat does not drift down on top of the person in the water. If he is not able to help in his rescue because of injury or unconsciousness, then place the boat one boat length upwind of the person and float down a rubber raft with a rescuer aboard to him. Carefully secure the raft to the mother vessel first and make sure the rescuer is wearing a Class I approved life vest. The two people can then be hauled back to the parent vessel. Rarely, if ever, should a second person go in the water to help the injured party. This is likely to create two people in need of rescue. Small boats can be maneuvered up to the injured party, preferably downwind of them, and rescue made, but larger sailboats and powerboats are more likely to injure or kill the person in the water as they rise and fall with enormous force. They are also more difficult to maneuver because the helmsman cannot see someone in the water close aboard.

Once the injured party has been maneuvered to the side of the boat, immediately pass a line formed in a large loop (about three feet in diameter) over his head. Use a bowline knot to secure the loop. Pass the line over his shoulders and up under his arms. Tension on the line will now bring the line securely up against the person's back and underarms. It can be further secured with a second line in front of the chest or by tying the loop tighter with a bight of its own line. If the bitter end of this line is secured to the boat, then the person is attached to the boat even if he loses his grip or slips when he tries to come aboard. If conditions are calm, then he can be brought aboard over the transom on the swim ladder. If there is a significant seaway, this will be dangerous. Under these circumstances, use a main halyard or a three-part hoist to haul him aboard. It is preferable to use the victim's safety harness as a point of attachment to haul him aboard. If he is not wearing one, then pass a line around his waist or use his belt as an additional fixation point for the haul. A line between the belt and the loop under his arms will distribute the load and can be used to attach the halyard. This will be easier on the person being hauled aboard. The rescuers should do most of the work in bringing the person aboard. The person in the water should conserve most of his strength to assist with tying the lines to himself. Otherwise, he is likely to exhaust his strength and be unable to assist in the process. The commercially available Lifesling can be used to haul the person aboard if he can get himself into it.

**Powerboat Procedures.** Man-overboard procedures for the powerboat operator are described in an internal training memorandum distributed to the U.S. Coast Guard Auxiliary. The procedure described is generally excellent, but I will make suggestions for changes that may improve one's chances for a successful recovery. The pamphlet separates the procedure into initial actions, actions to be taken if time permits, and approaches to the victim.

Initial actions are quite standard. Yell "Man overboard" as loudly as you can. Throw anything that floats into the water toward the victim. Then point at the victim, never taking your eyes off him. I would suggest continuing to scream "Man overboard" as loudly as you can until you are sure that you are heard. If you have not been heard, then run to the helm to alert the helmsman.

The person at the helm immediately should note his course on the compass and then turn the boat in a 180-degree turn to head back toward the victim. If you do not note your course, it may be very difficult to plot a return course. If your boat is equipped with Loran C, push the memory button to mark your position. Six or more short blasts of the horn will alert other boats in the area that you are making an emergency turn to pick up an overboard person.

If you are unable to locate the person in the water, fix your position and transmit an emergency message over the radio. The Coast Guard Auxiliary recommends using the message "Pan, Pan, Pan" followed by your distress call. They point out that "Mayday" is used when your boat is in danger. I strongly and completely disagree. The Mayday message is clearly understood as an emergency message by nearly everyone on the water. A person's life is in imminent danger and I believe that a Mayday call is proper and more effective. I seriously doubt that anyone would criticize its use under these circumstances.

At this point I believe that the information gathered by the Safety at Sea Committee should be added to the Coast Guard Auxiliary's recommendations. If the person in the water is spotted, I would recommend approaching the person slowly until you are two boat lengths away. If he is conscious, then carefully feed a Lifesling or a ring buoy with a long polypropylene line over the stern of your boat. Make sure the bitter end of the line is fastened securely to the stern. Then make a series of circles around the person until he can grasp the line or the buoy. You can then safely haul him to the side of the boat nearest the seas and wind (the windward side of the boat), so the boat is not likely to drift over him. At that point fasten a line around the victim as described earlier and fix this line to the boat. You may then haul him aboard using a block and tackle or two or more healthy crew mates.

If the victim is not conscious, then my first choice would be to maneuver next to him in relatively calm conditions. Again, I would prefer to maneuver the boat on the downwind (leeward) side of the victim so the boat does not drift over him. This is also the approach to be considered if there is only one or two crew left on board. If sea conditions are rough, the motion of the boat is unpredictable and recovery may not be possible. If your vessel is still fully manned, then position your vessel to windward of the victim and float down a seaworthy dinghy or inflatable life raft with a strong crewman aboard. This crew member should be wearing a life jacket and the dinghy or raft should be securely attached to the parent vessel with a strong line. Rescue may then be made more easily from the smaller vessel. This maneuver is usually not necessary if the parent vessel is under thirty feet in length.

## ON THE EDGE OF DISASTER

We thrashed through the storm. *Classic*'s stern rose and fell in a primitive rhythm, dancing to the syncopated beat of the twelve-foot seas. I was off watch and in the port bunk in the main cabin. Judy was at the wheel and Wayne was by her side. This was to be our first ocean passage. We all were innocents, pretending at knowledge and expertise we didn't have. All of us had experience in coastal passages, but that had not prepared us for these conditions. The crashing of our bow in the authoritative seas caused her to shudder with each thrust forward. Night had fallen two hours earlier. The squalls hid the lowered sky. Neither

Wayne nor Judy ventured to look beyond their south-westers except for quick, periodic surveys of our little world.

I lay there planning. We needed some rest. Perhaps I should heave to, but when I had tried it earlier, the boat's bow had run off before the wind like a frightened colt. Suddenly, I heard Judy's voice, harsh, alarmed, "Man overboard." We had joked about using the impersonal "Person overboard" in precruise planning, but now that the real thing confronted us, we clung to the familiar, the reliable—anything for God's sake, just HELP!

I don't think my feet even touched the cabin floor. I flew out into the cockpit, unaware of my own need for safety harness or even outer clothes. I only wore underwear while in my sleeping bag. Judy was hanging on to a yellow slickered arm which twisted this way and that with each boat motion. Al was now at my side and we both lunged for the body behind the arm. The three of us wrestled Wayne back into the cockpit. He had unclipped his harness, grasped the binnacle, and swung around it to take over the wheel from Judy. Then the boat dropped off a large wave and left him hanging in midair. When he caught up with the boat, he was overboard and only a superhuman effort allowed him to grab the stern rail. The sudden twisting impact of that landing had pulled out his right shoulder. He had hung on with his left.

Wayne was a powerfully built man, stocky, and in excellent physical condition. His right arm now hung uselessly at his side. He had dislocated the shoulder. We laid him down on a cockpit seat, his head and shoulders in Judy's lap. I knew that if I didn't reduce the dislocation quickly, his powerful muscles would go into spasm and we would never be able to get the job done without anesthesia at a hospital. I took his wrist in both my hands, put my wet, stockinged feet under his armpit and slowly and gently pulled, gradually bringing the limb up to 90 degrees from his side. It slipped back into the socket. We tucked Wayne into his bunk and then I shook and shook. The chances of finding him at night in a storm were remote at best. Thank God it all worked out!

# 2. Injuries and Their Management

The guiding principle for treating all injuries is to prevent further damage and to do whatever is necessary to allow the body's marvelous healing powers to assert themselves. This means that, whenever there is a question of a serious injury such as trauma to the neck or back or a broken bone with deformity, immobilizing the parts of the body on all sides of the wounded area can make the difference between permanent damage or death and a serious injury that will heal. This, in general, must take precedence over transferring the victim to a motorboat or vehicle for transport to a hospital. The only exception has to be when the injured person's position will expose him to further injury.

The major characteristic of all injuries is that they cause bruising under the skin and in the tissues accompanied by bleeding from small blood vessels and swelling of the tissues caused by fluid leaking from damaged tissues. In general, early elevation of the injured part will decrease the pressure within the injured vessels and tissues and lessen the swelling. Applying cold or iced compresses to the injured area will cause the blood vessels to contract and thereby decrease the bleeding (and its accompanying black and blue color). This will also help to decrease the swelling. Never apply heat to an injured part. This will only worsen the injury. The only exception to this is a charley horse (a cramped muscle). This may occur when you twist or turn the wrong way or are exposed to cold. It is not really an injury. A cramped muscle will relax when warmed and this will help bring relief.

It is okay to apply mild heat to an injured part three to five days after an injury to help relieve associated muscular cramping and to increase the blood supply to the area to clean up black and blue areas and reduce swelling. At this point, no harm is likely to be caused by the heat. With serious injuries such as fractures, however, this is still not a good idea and rest, ice, and elevation may properly be used for one to two weeks following the injury.

## PENETRATING INJURIES

A puncture wound (such as from a nail) should, in general, be treated by soaking the injured part in very warm to hot fresh water (without causing a burn) for at least a half-hour four times a day for three days. If the patient has not had a tetanus booster within the previous five years, he should be transported to a hospital for immunization. Any sign of infection (pain, redness, or swelling) indicates the need for professional help and antibiotics. More drastic treatment is, on occasion, needed under these circumstances and the patient should be under medical supervision.

Fishhooks are a common source of problems for the boating public. When the hook is well embedded, it is not possible to withdraw it backwards. It must be driven on through the tissues. Cut the eye off the hook with a pair of wire cutters. Then take a pair of pliers and push the hook through in the same direction that it entered. Try to follow the curve of the hook. When the tip appears at the skin, grasp it with a second pair of pliers and pull the rest through. Finally, soak the injured part in warm to hot water or apply hot packs. Treat as an infected wound (see infections below).

## LACERATIONS (CUTS)

The most appropriate thing to do for lacerations is to gently clean them out with warm fresh water and mild soap. Rinsing the wound out afterward with fresh water will remove debris, dirt, dead skin, and other possible sources of infection. The edges of the wound can be cleaned with an antiseptic such as Betadine solution or surgical scrub. The wound itself should not.

Most small lacerations can simply be covered with a small sterile adhesive bandage after cleaning. If they are small, they do not require suturing unless they are in an important cosmetic or functional area such as the eyelid. If the edges are separated by a gap of 1/4 inch or so, they can be held together with tape or butterfly adhesive bandages. If the wound is gaping widely and is deep, professional help must be sought and an effort made to determine whether important blood vessels, nerves, or tendons have been cut. Suturing must also be considered. It is still appropriate to cleanse the wound as described above and cover it with a sterile dressing before transporting the patient to a hospital. This will help to prevent further infection.

## STAB WOUNDS

A stab wound in the chest or abdomen should be examined promptly by a physician. Even though the entry wound may be small, serious internal injury could have occurred. Open chest wounds should be sealed with plastic film (such as a plastic grocery store wrap) and large sterile

pads. These can be secured with adhesive tape. Open
abdominal wounds with the contents protruding are also
best covered with plastic film and a sterile pad. The
abdomen can then be splinted with a sheet wrapped
around the patient's body and strapped with adhesive or
pinned in position. Both situations require emergency
medical evacuation.

## CRUSH INJURIES

Crush injuries frequently happen to commercial fishermen and, on occasion, to boaters. A sailor's finger or hand
can get caught in a winch or haul. The person's skin is
often broken or pulled off and bones may be fractured.
After freeing the injured person, lay him in a berth with
warm blankets. Treat him for shock by laying him flat and
propping his legs up on some pillows. This increases the
blood supply to the important vital centers of the body.
Control bleeding as necessary. Wash the wounds with soap
and water and cover with a sterile dressing. If the skin is
badly mauled, treat it like a severe burn with silver sulfadiazine cream spread over the split skin and apply sterile
gauze. Elevate the injured part with a sling or pillows and
apply cold compresses or an ice bag. Give the victim some
pain medication and start antibiotics, if you have them
available. Keflex 500 mg four times a day would be my
choice. If a part has been amputated, save it in a refrigerator, but do not freeze. Cold, fresh water with a little
salt added (1 tsp per 8 oz glass of water) will help preserve
the part. Get help and medevac fast. This is a Mayday
emergency! The amputated part should be taken to the
hospital along with the victim. It may be able to be
resutured to the body.

## BLEEDING

Major bleeding from a wound requires direct compression with a gauze pad and your weight pushing down on the pad *hard* for a minimum of ten minutes (for venous bleeding) and thirty minutes or longer for arterial bleeding (it spurts). Avoid peeking to see if the bleeding has stopped. Keep pressure applied long after the bleeding has been controlled by using a pressure bandage. Leave on the original gauze pad and apply new ones over it. Bind it with a firm dressing. Don't worry about cleaning the wound. Just get the injured person to professional help *after* you get the bleeding controlled. Most major bleeding can be controlled this way. Very occasionally, it may be lifesaving to apply a tourniquet, but this should be reserved for amputations or other catastrophic situations. The tourniquet must be applied tightly enough to shut off the arterial pressure as well as the venous or it will not work. Take a piece of cloth and tie it loosely around the injured limb above the point of injury or amputation. Place a stick, a screwdriver, or a similar item under the tie and twist it again and again. This will apply a controllable amount of pressure to the entire limb within the cloth. Apply more turns until the bleeding stops. Obviously, prompt medical help must be obtained and a medical evacuation should be arranged.

## SHOCK

Shock, which can be thought of as a poor supply of blood to the body, is due to poor circulation of the blood. Visible signs of shock include a cold, clammy, pallid skin, rapid pulse (90 beats or more per minute), and rapid respirations (20 or more breaths per minute). This can be caused by blood loss, severe pain, or heart failure.

If the source of the blood loss can be seen, stop it. Use pressure and bulky dressings held by a firmly applied elastic bandage or adhesive tape. If the bleeding is in the abdomen or chest, then outside help will be immediately needed. Shock from severe pain results in pooling of the blood in the small vessels all over the body. This is caused by a paralysis of the muscular walls of these blood vessels. The lack of tone in the vessel walls means that the heart doesn't get the blood back from the body to pump it out again. Treatment at the scene for both types of problems requires the following: lay the patient down flat; elevate his feet and legs above his head about one to two feet on pillows; apply elastic bandages to his legs from the toes up to squeeze blood from these extremities to the central core of the body.

If the source of shock is heart failure, the patient cannot be allowed to lie flat. This will only increase his difficulty in breathing. He has no shortage of blood to be conserved, only a weakness in the heart muscle and an inability to move that blood. This patient should be allowed to sit up with his back against some pillows. Heart strengthening medications such as digitalis and diuretics will be needed. Any patient showing evidence of shock is a Mayday emergency. Get him to a hospital fast!

### DISLOCATIONS

The basic first aid principle for dislocations and fractures is to "splint it where it lies." By doing this, you will stabilize the injured part and prevent further injury. In general, it is preferable to apply a support to the dislocated part and to transport the patient to a medical facility. If you were to attempt to reduce the dislocation, injury to adjacent nerve structures could result in paralysis of the limb.

## FRACTURES

Simple fractures may not have to be set as an emergency. They can be taken care of a day or two later with little change in the ultimate result. Simply splint and protect the broken part from further injury until you can get medical assistance. The principle of splinting is to make sure that the injured part is supported by a sturdy, uninjured portion of the body which is not subject to motion. Spare pieces of wood protected by a padding of cloth may be used. Have the splint extend as far as possible up the uninjured portion of the injured limb as well as beyond the area of injury and bind it well to the uninjured portions. Again, rest, ice, and elevation are often helpful. Fractures of a finger or toe can often be splinted by taping the injured digit to an adjacent uninjured finger or toe.

Compound fractures in which the bone has broken through the skin are very dangerous. The wound should be carefully washed with soap and fresh water and rinsed. The wound should then be covered with sterile bandages. The part must be splinted carefully to prevent the broken ends of the bone from cutting important nerves. Finally, immediate transport to a hospital will be needed and should be professionally arranged if possible.

## SPINAL CORD INJURIES

A person who has injuries to the spine or neck should be immobilized with a long board (such as a door) with padding for the small of the back. Move the patient as a unit, preferably with several people handling each part and rolling him over onto the board rather than lifting him. Neck injuries are critical and the neck of a person who has such an injury must not be moved at all.* Immobilize the patient's neck with a brace made of rolled towels and move him with a long board to a hospital. Again, professional assistance with transportation to the hospital can be critical.

## HEAD INJURIES

Head injuries are assessed on a clinical basis by the results of the injury. If the person was hurt or stunned but not knocked out, he did not, most likely, sustain a serious injury. Treat him with ice to the injured area. The patient should be carefully questioned to determine if he can remember exactly what happened to him and what occurred after the injury. Any memory loss may indicate a concussion. In this case, you should still treat with ice to the injured area, but in addition get a medical evaluation performed as soon as possible.

Late bleeding inside the head days or weeks after a head injury can occur, with headaches increasing in severity. This should cause you to seek medical help. If the injured party lost consciousness or is confused, then the possibility of a serious injury must be considered. Put the patient to bed with ice and seek help as soon as possible. If the patient is unconscious, put him in a secure berth so he can't injure himself further, and make sure he is able to breathe without difficulty. Keep his head straight and do not allow his neck to flex sharply (such as can be caused

---

*A broken neck (or fractured cervical vertebra) can damage the spinal cord at a spot which may result in paralysis of both arms and legs.

by a pillow). Bending the head forward allows the tongue to obstruct breathing. Obviously, immediate medical assistance must be obtained and medical evacuation sought.

## BURNS

Ordinary burns are classified according to severity. If the burn is superficial, it simply hurts and the skin is reddened, but undamaged. This is a first-degree burn. If the skin is blistered and the underlying deeper layers of the skin are still intact, but the outer layer is damaged, this is a second-degree burn. If the skin is denuded, burned white or black, or completely burned off leaving underlying fat or muscle showing, then the burn is most serious and is called a third-degree burn.

All burns should be cleansed with mild soap and fresh water. Remove any visible foreign body with a forceps or wash off with the water. Minor burns can simply be placed under cold running water or in cold compresses for thirty minutes to an hour. This will help to relieve the pain and diminish swelling. Then apply a petroleum jelly gauze dressing.

A second-degree burn should also be cleansed as described above. Blisters should be left intact, however, since they help to seal off the raw tissues underneath from infection.

Major burns should be handled as follows: remove the patient from the source of the fire. If his clothing is afire, roll him in a blanket to snuff out the flames. At a calm anchorage, jumping overboard may be an option, but this should not be attempted in a seaway. Buckets of cold seawater can assist in putting out the flames. Fire extinguishers should be available but these must not be aimed at a person, only at the source of the fire. When the fire is out, all burned clothing should be removed unless it is stuck to the skin. Burns should be cleaned with soap and water and may be coated with an antibacterial cream such as silver sulfadiazine. A sterile gauze can be placed over the cream and fixed in place with a roller gauze or elastic bandage. Large burns should be covered with sterile plastic film rather than petroleum jelly gauze. Lacking this supply, applying silver sulfadiazine cream and plastic food wrap is a reasonable substitute. Immediate transportation to a medical facility is necessary since antibiotics and possible skin grafting may be needed.

Burns around the eyes, nose, or mouth require special attention, since burning gasses could affect vision or may have entered the respiratory tract and could cause difficulty in breathing later on. Get to a hospital.

Chemical burns should be flushed with water. No effort at neutralizing an acid with a base or vice versa should be made. The heat from such reactions may increase damage to the skin.

## IMMERSION INJURIES

Immersion (or trench foot) injuries result from the prolonged exposure of the feet to cold and dampness at temperatures above freezing. There is usually prolonged immobility in damp or wet boots or sneakers. The cold and numbness associated with this is initially well tolerated. Upon return to the warm cabin, however, the injured person experiences severe burning, pain, and associated swelling and redness of the feet. Often, when severe, the feet are pale or waxy and bluish in color. Warming of the foot produces redness. Blisters may occur with swelling or edema. Ulcerations and gangrene (local tissue death) may result. Treatment should be bed rest, elevation of the leg or legs to minimize the swelling, wrapping of the feet and legs in cotton followed by wool. Warm the central areas of the body such as the torso as well as the hands and head. Keep local heat away from the damaged feet to avoid further damage to the injured skin.

## FROSTBITE

Freezing of tissues exposed to subfreezing temperatures will result in frostbite. Fingers, toes, ears, and the nose are commonly affected. Similar in results to a burn, the damage can be analogous. Mild frostbite will result in the extremity becoming white or pale and numb. Rewarming of the affected part results in pins and needles or a tingling sensation. Gradual rewarming of the affected part is recommended. No other special treatment is needed. Greater sensitivity to the cold will result from this injury. Moderate frostbite will result in blister formation and cause loss of the surface skin. Rapid rewarming of the central body and gentle rewarming of the affected extremity in lukewarm water is suggested. Bring the injured person to an emergency room for further treatment. Antibiotics may be needed.

## HYPOTHERMIA

Hypothermia is caused by loss of body heat due to prolonged exposure to the elements or to the water. It can result in a loss of motor and/or sensory function in the injured person. It can cause unconsciousness and arrhythmias of the heart. Institute cardiopulmonary resuscitation (CPR) if appropriate (see chapter 4). Remove all clothes. Dry the person with a soft towel. Redress in warm dry clothes. Wrap in a blanket. If he is conscious, give him warm liquids to drink. In extreme cases use other people's bodies to help warm the hypothermic person. Do not give alcohol as this dilates the peripheral blood vessels and increases heat loss. Do not immerse in hot water. Warm the patient gradually.

## SKIN INFECTIONS

Infections of the surface of the body can occur in almost any location. They can involve pimples on the forehead to infected cuts on the fingers, abscesses of the breast to infected teeth. Certain general principles apply to all infections.

To recognize infection, you should note any of the following characteristics: redness, swelling, pain, or drainage. Any two of the preceding are hallmarks of infection. Often a fever with chills or sweating may also occur, but this usually happens when the infection has invaded the body to deeper areas than just the surface.

Treatment of infection involves the following: Whenever possible apply heat to the area. Heat increases the blood supply to the infected area and this brings more white blood cells to the site. These white blood cells attack the invading bacteria and are the body's first defense. If a finger or toe is infected, soak the infected part in hot water. It should be as hot as the person can stand without causing his skin to blister. Gradually warm it up and have him keep dipping the digit in and out to allow him to tolerate the heat. Frequently, the bacteria are heat sensitive and you can interfere with their life cycle as well as bring more blood to the area. Infected gums may be treated with warm to hot mouthwashes, using either a mixture of astringent mouthwash (such as Lavoris) and hot water or plain hot water. Soaking or rinsing should be done as often as possible—preferably for twenty to thirty minutes four times a day.

Similarly, a breast abscess can be treated with warm packs applied to the infected breast for thirty to sixty minutes four times a day. One way to do this is to fill a cloth bag or towel with sand. Dampen the cloth or use wet sand and warm in the oven for fifteen minutes on low heat. Alternatively, leave an ice bag or other container with water on the engine while running it to get it to just about the right temperature. Hot water bottles can also be used. Do not burn the skin! Test the warm pack with your hand or wrist first.

If the person not only shows local symptoms such as pain, redness, and swelling in the infected part, but also begins to show signs of generalized body reactions (fever, sweating, chills, or red streaks radiating away from the original infection), then get medical help. Generally, these infections are due to surface type bacteria such as streptococcus or staphylococcus. These "bugs" are best treated with antibiotics, so shorten your cruise and take the person to a doctor. A day without antibiotics while an infection becomes established can turn an easily treatable problem into a life-threatening one. Infections should be treated vigorously and early. They should *never* be ignored! If an abscess develops, it may be necessary to drain it to gain relief. See your doctor or the local hospital.

# 3. Medical Problems from Head to Toe

## THE EYE

**Eye Injuries.** The eyes are our connection to reality. We are so accustomed to trusting what we see that, if we suddenly are denied access to that sense, we are immobilized, unable to function, and may even wish for death. No other loss has such a devastating effect on an individual as the loss of sight. For these reasons, we should take special care of our eyes. Whenever an injury or infection occurs, take it seriously and treat it properly and promptly.

Eye injuries are often caused by a foreign body (piece of metal, sand, etc.) getting in the eye. It is very important *not* to try to wipe out or pick out the foreign body. You will risk seriously damaging the cornea or surface of the eye by doing so. This would distort or cloud vision in the future. Try to irrigate the eye with sterile water or saline, or at least clean, fresh water. Have the person lie down and gently part the lids with your second and third fingers. Flush the eye softly by pouring the water directly on it. You may be able to wash the foreign body out. If not, leave it there. Patch the eye, or even both eyes if you have enough help to guide the injured person. Take the injured one to an ophthalmologist or at least to the emergency room of the local hospital. Antibiotic ointment and patching are often all that is needed, but careful assessment by a professional is essential. Topical antibiotic eye medications such as gentamicin eye drops or Neosporin ophthalmic ointment applied to the injured eye before patching may improve comfort and minimize infection while the patient awaits medical assistance. If there is any question that the eyeball was cut or that a foreign body actually entered into the eye (as opposed to lying on the surface), then immediate evaluation by an ophthalmologist is mandatory and medical evacuation should be arranged. Until he can be seen, the patient should lie with both eyes patched and with his head slightly elevated.

Chemical burns to the eye are often due to acids or alkalis. Treat by *immediately* irrigating the eye with water. Hold the eye open under a steady stream of fresh water and irrigate continuously for at least five minutes. If an alkali comes in contact with the eye, irrigate even longer, perhaps a minimum of ten minutes. Evaluation in an emergency room, which will include testing of the eye with pH paper, is then warranted.

Blunt trauma to the eye such as can be caused by a block or boom should be treated with cold compresses or ice. Bleeding inside the eye may occur and result in high intraocular pressures. Evaluation in an emergency room should be obtained. Eleven percent of people with blunt trauma have a significant eye injury, and all should be examined by an ophthalmologist.

**Eye Infections.** Infections of the eye are characterized by redness and tears in the white area (sclera) and the inside of the lids. Often a crusty debris will be found just under the edge of the lid. Redness with a purulent discharge is due to a bacterial infection. This is called conjunctivitis, but the name is unimportant. Local treatment with warm packs is helpful. Your eye doctor is likely to recommend antibiotic drops or ointment. I would suggest seeing at least a local family practitioner. Neosporin or other antibiotic ophthalmic (eye) drops or ointment such as gentamicin drops may be suggested. They can be placed in the eye three or four times a day for at least five days. You may (but do not have to) patch the affected eye for a day. External eye inflammation can be caused by bacteria, viruses, and allergy. The diagnosis is often hard without special examining tools. It is considered safe to use an antibiotic ointment or drops until an examination can be performed.

**Red Eye.** Pain in the eye itself with redness is a much more serious problem and requires urgent medical assistance. A red, painful eye, with some loss of vision and a small pupil indicates an "iritis." This requires an ophthalmologist's evaluation and advice. A painful eye that is sensitive to light or aches must also be seen promptly. Initial treatment is local antibiotic ointment or drops as above; patch the eye and, if possible, have the patient rest in his bunk until professional help can be obtained.

**Viral Infections.** If a red, painful eye occurs with clear tears only, then a viral infection must be suspected. This can, at times, be due to herpes simplex and can lead to severe eye injury. An ophthalmologist must be consulted promptly. He may recommend an antiviral agent called I.D.U. (idoxuridine).

**Subconjunctival Hemorrhage.** A bright, red eye without pain may simply be a subconjunctival hemorrhage (bleeding just below the surface of the membrane). This usually resolves on its own, but the patient should be evaluated by an ophthalmologist.

**Infected or Blocked Tear Duct.** Tears with severe pain just lateral to (or to the side of) the bridge of the nose is caused by an obstruction or infection of the tear duct. Hot compresses and antibiotics will be effective, but often an ophthalmologist can relieve the pain quickly by probing the duct and releasing the pressure.

**Sty.** Redness and pain and swelling of the lid (a sty) can be treated with very warm compresses and an antibiotic eye drop or ointment. If the eye is not responsive to local treatment in twenty-four hours, the patient may need antibiotics by mouth.

**Contact Lens Injuries.** Contact lenses may cause corneal abrasions (scratching of the membrane of the eye) if they are left on too long. Prolonged use of contact lenses may cause pain up to four hours later. Apply an antibiotic eye drop or ointment, patch the eye or both eyes for twenty-four hours, and consult an ophthalmologist. Do not use the contacts again until an eye doctor has been able to determine whether they are causing damage to your eye. When patching an eye, take an eye pad, fold it in half, and apply it to the closed lid. Then, take a second eye pad and apply it open to the first pad and secure with cellophane tape.

**Eye Allergies.** Irritations can be due to eye allergies to cat fur, pollens, and other substances. The best approach is to (a) remove the source of the irritation (for example, wash your hands after handling a cat), (b) take an oral antihistamine such as Benadryl 25 mg once or perhaps twice in twelve hours (this may cause some sleepiness), and (c) for more persistent problems that will not resolve, see an ophthalmologist.

**Glaucoma.** Most patients who develop glaucoma have no pain or blurring. For this reason, everyone over forty years of age should be checked with a pressure test every two years. Blurring of vision or narrowing of your field of vision can be a late sign of glaucoma. This is increased fluid pressure within the eye. Its best treatment is prevention. If you are over the age of forty or have a family history of glaucoma, see an ophthalmologist and have a pressure test done. Treatment is to decrease the pressure in the eye. Certain eye drops recommended by your eye doctor are commonly used. Laser treatments and surgery are occasionally needed.

Severe eye pain with a loss of vision is often due to acute narrow angle glaucoma, a sudden form of glaucoma. Nausea and vomiting may be prominent symptoms and are due to the pain. Immediate treatment in an emergency room is mandatory.

**Retinal Problems.** Retinal detachment is a disease in which, due to degeneration or injury, the lining tissue inside the back of the eye (retina) separates from the layer behind it. This tears the connections with the nerves and blood supply and interferes with vision. It causes loss of a field or area of vision. Often, a bright flash of light within the eye and the appearance of floating specks herald the onset of the detachment. Treatment is difficult even under the best of circumstances and the best you can do on a boat is to have the person lie down with the head slightly elevated and patch both eyes. The patient should avoid jumping, running, heavy work, or excitement; he should stay quiet to prevent further detachment and seek medical assistance as soon as possible. Loss of vision in an eye should be considered an emergency until proven otherwise and demands medical evacuation. Retinal artery occlusion, retinal hemorrhage, and retinal detachment are all possible causes.

**Medical Diseases Affecting the Eye.** Diabetes, arteriosclerosis, and tumors can all affect the eyes. They seldom cause an emergency problem, however, and require professional care in a proper setting. Chronic loss of vision is often seen in cataract formation and macular degeneration (loss of the photosensitive cells in the eye). These conditions often respond to surgery or other treatments.

**Brain Diseases Affecting the Eye.** Double vision sometimes means that internal disease in the brain is occurring. If it is accompanied by severe headache, then a ruptured intracerebral aneurysm (a blown out artery in the brain) may be occurring. Immediate medical evacuation is mandatory.

## THE EAR

Ears are subject to infections, foreign bodies, and blockage from wax. Punctured eardrums from diving are also potentially a problem.

**Ear Infections.** Ear infections can be external or internal. External ear infection in which the ear feels itchy and scratchy and irritated may be due to swimming or diving and is treated with antibiotic eardrops. Any neomycin, polymyxin B, hydrocortisone eardrop mixture is acceptable. Use two or three times a day until the symptoms have gone; usually this takes at least five days. A cotton wad will hold the drops in. Do not swim or dive for at least a week after the symptoms have disappeared or they may return.

Internal ear infections are characterized by pain in the ear. Drainage from the ear is a late sign and indicates that treatment should have been started earlier. The patient should see a doctor, who will recommend an appropriate antibiotic—probably ampicillin 500 mg three or four times a day depending on the size of the person or erythromycin 500 mg four times a day. Keflex 500 mg three times per day may also be considered. Treatment should be continued with an effective antibiotic for at least one week. As with external ear infections, the patient shouldn't swim or dive for at least four weeks after the symptoms have disappeared. Ear infections that have been inadequately treated can lead to mastoiditis, an infection of the mastoid sinuses in the bone behind the ear. This can lead to a brain abscess and is a threat to life. Ear infections should not be ignored and professional medical advice should be sought, proper cultures taken, and appropriate treatment instituted.

**Diver's Ear.** Scuba diving can lead to punctured eardrums. If the ear has been unable to equalize the pressure between the outside water pressure and the internal air environment, the delicate membrane that transmits the sound waves from the air to the tiny bones that send it to the inner ear is broken. This can occur if the tiny tubes that connect the inner ear with the back of the throat are blocked. That sometimes happens when you have a cold. Rule one here is, don't dive if you have a cold, cough, or sinusitis. The symptoms of a ruptured eardrum are pain in the ear and, sometimes, bleeding from the inside of the ear. As with an ear infection, you should treat diver's ear with antibiotics; swimming or diving should be avoided until the patient gets professional advice from an otolaryngologist (ear, nose, and throat or "ENT" doctor). During recuperation, not only should the ear be kept dry, but the patient should avoid blowing his nose, which could transmit infection to the middle ear via the eustachian tube. A ruptured eardrum can also occur from a slapping injury to the ear or, on occasion, by a fall while waterskiing. The recommendation is that no water should be allowed in the ear until an ENT doctor tells you that the eardrum has healed.

Ringing in the ear after diving or dizziness immediately after diving is considered an ENT emergency. It may indicate a rupture in the round window membrane or a perilymphatic fistula which can lead to complete deafness or permanent loss of balance. Seek professional help immediately if this occurs.

**Foreign Bodies.** Foreign bodies such as insects, marbles, or peas are very difficult to extract without proper instruments. An insect should be drowned in mineral oil prior to attempting an extraction. If you can see it and grab it with a pair of forceps, do so. If not, be careful that you don't push it in even farther while trying to remove it. Careful irrigation may be of help here. You may, however, require professional assistance. Children are the ones most prone to this problem.

Wax is, by far, the most common ear complaint. Hearing becomes more distant, pressure builds within the ear, and the person can't hear at all for several hours after swimming. Simply take warm water and irrigate the ear. If this is not effective, dry the external ear with some cotton and drop in hydrogen peroxide drops two or three times a day and keep the stuff in with a wad of cotton. Debrox or Murine eardrops are also wax softeners and may be used. This will break up the wax. The person shouldn't be concerned at the crackling, bubbling noise heard when putting these drops in the ear. After two or three days, the wax can then be easily irrigated from the ear with warm water either by your doctor or by yourself. This last step must be done or the wax will cake up in the ear and make it more difficult to remove.

Irrigation of the ear is performed with a syringe. Usually a bulb syringe, such as an Asepto syringe, is used, but a good size (20–50 cc) piston syringe may be a reasonable substitute. Ear syringes are available at many pharmacies. Warm water that is comfortable to the wrist is placed in a container. The water is drawn into the syringe and gently flushed into the ear. The patient may hold his head sideways over a sink to catch the drainage. The ear should not be obstructed by the top of the syringe, nor should the syringe actually enter the ear canal. The canal should be flushed repeatedly with warm water; hot water should be added gradually to make the solution warmer. It should at all times be comfortable to the patient. After a number of irrigations, pieces of wax will begin to come out, and, when a large plug is flushed from the ear, the irrigation may be stopped. It usually takes four or five quarts of warm water to complete the irrigation. At no time should the patient experience pain. If he does, the irrigation should be discontinued.

### THE NOSE

**Infections.** Infection within the nose is either the result of external injury (uncommon) or internal injury due to a probing finger. Infection is associated with pain in the nose. It is potentially very dangerous since there are no protective lymph nodes to drain and block the spread of infection in the nose. The result is that, if the external barriers are broken down, infection can be transmitted directly into the blood vessels of the brain. This can be fatal. If pain due to an infection in the nose occurs, early treatment with erythromycin 500 mg by mouth three times per day or ampicillin 500 mg four times per day for a minimum of five days should be used. A doctor should be consulted.

**Bleeding.** Similarly a bloody nose is usually due to an external injury or the probing finger. It can sometimes be quite excessive and frightening. It should not be more serious than that, however, unless the patient has a bleeding tendency. It can be a sign of high blood pressure. It should be treated by cold compresses, and direct pressure on the nose. The patient should sit down and rest with his head elevated. Occasionally the nose will have to be packed. A single long roll of narrow petroleum jelly gauze can be unrolled and gently inserted into the affected nostril with a pair of smooth forceps or a needle-nose pliers and pushed upward until it will advance no further. More packing is placed until no more will fit in the nose. This packing should be left for at least four to six hours.

**Fractures.** A broken nose will occur from direct trauma. The nose need not be set immediately unless there is an obvious deformity. Cold compresses and pain medications may be taken. Medical assessment at the emergency room is advisable, since early manipulation is, at times, helpful.

### THE CHEST

Chest and respiratory problems can run the gamut from the common cold to heart attacks. We will discuss each in its place.

**The Common Cold.** The common cold, characterized by sneezing and coughing, is usually not associated with a fever. If the temperature is over 101°F, you may be dealing with a more serious illness. Treat the common cold with loads of fluids, rest, and patience. Vitamin C has been recommended as helpful by some, in doses up to five grams every six hours. Although this has not been clinically proven, there are numerous anecdotal stories praising its effectiveness. If a severe sore throat is present, then antibiotics may be needed. Early use of antibiotics may prevent the complications from strep throat, including rheumatic fever and nephritis. A visit to the doctor will allow for throat cultures, chest X rays, and blood tests (if needed), and the doctor will determine which antibiotic would be most effective for you. Penicillin or ampicillin are frequently recommended.

**Cough.** A mild cough of short duration and without more serious symptoms does not usually require treatment. Certainly the patient should not smoke (if he or she is so afflicted). Cough drops or a cough syrup such as Phenergan expectorant may be helpful here. Cough syrups containing codeine are more effective, but make the patient sleepy; they should only be used at bedtime.

A deep cough, especially one in which a lot of phlegm is brought up, must be treated with antibiotics. For respiratory infections, choices include ampicillin 500 mg by mouth four times a day, erythromycin 500 mg by mouth four times a day, or perhaps tetracycline, 250 mg four times a day. Keflex 500 mg by mouth three or four times a day may also be used. Your doctor's advice on this should be sought, since the choice of antibiotic will depend on his experience with similar illnesses that season. He may have found that a particular antibiotic has been very effective this year. You can benefit from his experience. A particular antibiotic should not be used if the patient has a known allergy to that class of antibiotics (for example, penicillin allergy should eliminate ampicillin from the options). In all cases, antibiotics for respiratory infections should be continued a minimum of seven and up to ten days. A cough syrup such as Phenergan expectorant with codeine (one tablespoon every four hours) can give tremendous relief and may allow sleep. If the patient coughs up blood, a more serious process may be going on. Put him to bed and get help.

**Wheezing.** Wheezing, with or without a dry cough, is often a sign of asthma. It is caused by an allergic reaction to allergens in the air. The bronchial tubes leading to the lungs react to the allergen by going into spasm. As their diameter contracts, it becomes more difficult for the patient to breathe. As hard as it is to breathe in, it is even harder to breathe out. If you listen to the patient breathe, his expiration is prolonged and you may hear a wheeze or wheezes as he breathes out. Wheezing is treated by using a bronchodilator to open up the tubes going to the lungs, allowing the person to breathe more easily. For acute spasm, a Ventolin Inhaler or Bronkaid Mist inhaler is used three or four times during the day, while for maintenance treatment, Slo-Phyllin 250 mg by mouth four times per day will handle the usual case. Very severe cases of asthma seldom occur without a prior history of the disease so the patient will probably have some medications with him. If you have severe asthma—or a crew member does—it may be a wise precaution to have a syringe or two of epinephrine aboard in case a really extreme situation occurs and you are concerned that someone may die. Then an injection with a tiny amount (0.1 cc) of 1:1000 epinephrine every minute (up to 0.5 cc) until the symptoms are relieved will help the problem. If this is a situation that applies to you, you should get specific instructions from your doctor in advance because of the variables that occur from patient to patient.

Asthma can come on suddenly and become severe quickly. If you are prone to this affliction, always bring your asthma medication with you. Even a short day trip can put you out of reach of your doctor or hospital. Primatene tablets and Bronkaid Mist might be carried for such a situation by a skipper concerned about dealing with such an occurrence. Neither requires a prescription.

Wheezing, in association with a bad cough and a low-grade fever, in a patient not known to have asthma, may be a sign of asthmatic bronchitis and should be treated both with antibiotics and with Slo-Phyllin or inhaler. In the older age group with known heart problems, wheezing can be an early sign of heart failure, especially when associated with swelling of the feet and ankles during the day. This should alert one to getting early medical help.

**Chest Pain.** Chest pain is often frightening but not always serious. It should be evaluated calmly and thoughtfully. Is the pain made worse by taking a deep breath? If so, it is unlikely that the pain is a heart attack. It is more likely that this pain is due to a muscle spasm in the intercostal muscles (between the ribs). This usually lasts only a few minutes and disappears with rest. Have the patient breathe slowly and with measured rather than very deep breaths. Have him sit or lie down and rest. Stay with him and reassure him. He should be all right.

Similar pain, lasting longer (a day or more), is often referred to as pleurisy. If fever occurs with the pain, an antibiotic may be needed and you should seek medical assistance. If the pain is very severe *and* is associated with severe difficulty in breathing, the person may have had a pulmonary embolus or blood clot to the lung. Alternatively, he may have a spontaneous pneumothorax (a hole in the lung) causing air to escape into the space around the lung. Usually, people survive this kind of crisis, but prompt medical help can dramatically affect the outlook. Have the victim lie down propped up on two or three pillows, give him pain medication if you have this aboard. Obviously, this is a condition that requires professional assistance as soon as possible and a medical evacuation should be obtained.

**Heart Attacks.** Chest pain in the middle of the front of the chest, especially if it is a heavy weight, pressure, or squeezing pain, is often a warning of an impending heart attack. This might be associated with pain going into the left shoulder, arm, or even hand. If the pain lasts only a few minutes and is associated with hard work or fright, it may be angina—meaning that the heart is temporarily without enough oxygen and warning that it could be hurt if the person doesn't slow down. This is not usually a heart attack. The treatment is to sit or lie down and to try to consciously relax. The pain will go away with rest. The patient should not ignore this symptom or pretend that it isn't important or was just indigestion just because it has gone away. Instead, he should see a doctor immediately for an examination and advice. This step may prevent a heart attack! Nitroglycerin (one tablet) placed under the tongue will often be prescribed for patients with recurrent angina. Until the person has been checked out by a cardiologist, he should avoid as much stressful and heavy work as possible. Obviously such a warning means that he should be carefully evaluated as soon as possible.

If the pain is crushing and lasts more than fifteen minutes, it probably indicates that the patient is either having a heart attack or is at considerable risk of having one. Give him a nitroglycerin tablet as above if it is available. Repeat in five minutes if the pain has not gone. Have him lie down and give him pain medication if available. Immediate transfer to a hospital is necessary. This is a Mayday type of emergency, for early hospital treatment can prevent severe cardiac damage and may save a life. If the patient becomes unconscious, evaluate him for possible use of CPR (see chapter 4) by assessing the presence or absence of breathing and a pulse.

**Arrhythmias.** If a fluttering sensation is present in the chest with a markedly irregular pulse, then an arrhythmia (irregular heart rhythm) is present. This can decrease the effectiveness of the heart and may require medication. For sustained fluttering, treatment in a hospital will be needed and prompt evacuation is advised. A short episode of fluttering, lasting less than a minute or two, without dizziness, should be evaluated by a physician, but more electively.

A gradually increasing shortness of breath may indicate a gradual failing of the heart. It may be associated with swelling of the ankles that goes away when the patient sleeps (and his feet are up), but returns during the day. This, again, requires medical attention. A diuretic is usually prescribed.

An otherwise healthy person may suddenly develop apprehension, shortness of breath, weakness, and a discomfort in the chest. A fluttering in the chest may be noted and the heart may feel as if it is thumping like a hammer. Have the patient lie down and take his pulse. If the pulse is very rapid, say 150 or 200 beats per minute, feel the neck for the carotid pulse. If you feel just below the jaw in the space between the side of the Adam's apple and the neck muscles, you will feel a pulse. This is the carotid artery (see figure 3). Gentle pressure here for a few seconds will frequently break the rhythmic aberration and the

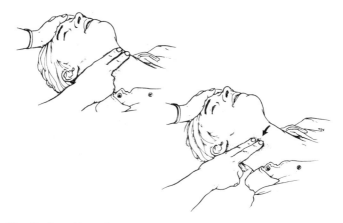

*Fig. 3. Locating the carotid pulse. From* Healthcare Provider's Manual for Basic Life Support, © *American Heart Association. Reproduced with permission.*

heart will slow right down. This maneuver should not be done on an elderly person since it could lead to a stroke. The patient should rest for a couple of hours. Make sure that the pulse does not speed up again. A person with this condition should, of course, be checked out by a doctor, who will use an EKG and other tests. Other types of arrhythmias are associated with heart disease and require specific medication. If you or any of your crew are prone to this, ask your cardiologist to give you some medication to use if an arrhythmia should occur.

If you are present when someone suddenly collapses and stops breathing, they may have had a sudden arrhythmia (irregular and inefficient heart action). Many lives can be saved by starting CPR immediately (see chapter 4).

**Fainting.** The conditions described above must be differentiated from a simple fainting spell. Factors leading to fainting are fatigue, anxiety, dehydration, hunger, pain, and blood loss. The person experiencing this problem becomes anxious and begins to perspire. His skin becomes pale and clammy and he may complain of dizziness. He will then lose consciousness and may appear close to death. His pulse will be very slow or unobtainable and his respirations shallow. He should be laid flat. This will restore blood supply to the brain and he will gradually awaken. He should be kept flat for an hour or so, or until he has fully regained his color, warmth, and alertness, or he may faint again. An attempt at correcting the factors that led to the fainting (such as dehydration) should be made.

## THE ABDOMEN

**Cramps and Diarrhea.** The best treatment for cramps and diarrhea is Imodium, which is available without a prescription. The sufferer should take two capsules initially, wait two hours, and, if cramps or diarrhea persist, take one capsule with each unformed movement. Usually, that will suffice. Alternative treatments might be Lomotil (available by prescription) one tablet after each movement (up to three a day) or four to eight tablespoons of Kaopectate every four hours.

If fever occurs with cramps and/or diarrhea, sweating and hot flashes, or feeling warm, the possibility of food poisoning should be considered. This may occur one to six hours after ingesting contaminated food or water. Eggs, mayonnaise, fish, and meats can become contaminated if improperly refrigerated. Medical attention is needed. Plenty of clear fluids should be taken (if they can be kept down) to counteract the dehydration of the diarrhea. Antibiotics may be needed. Tetracycline, erythromycin, or ampicillin may be used. Early consultation with your doctor is advisable, since antibiotics may mask a more serious condition. Stool cultures may be advised by the doctor since salmonella infections sometimes require longer-term treatment and because other organisms may be involved in resistant diarrhea. Lomotil or Imodium may offer comfort while the antibiotic is starting to have an effect.

Traveler's diarrhea (known in Mexican waters as Montezuma's revenge) is due to a number of infecting organisms in unsanitary water or from fresh vegetables or fruit contaminated with human waste. It is often recommended that a traveler who will be in such an area for a brief time (a week, perhaps) obtain doxycycline (Vibramycin) from his doctor and take 100 mg per day preventively. If the traveler will be there for a significantly longer period of time, then preventive medication is not advisable. Under such circumstances, treat supportively with fluids and medications for diarrhea as above until you can get the person to a doctor. If the symptoms persist, amebic dysentery may be present. Flagyl 750 mg three times a day is used for this. A doctor must be consulted to order appropriate tests.

**Constipation.** Unassociated with illness, but often causing discomfort, is constipation. This is a very common problem on boats. There is something about the movement of a boat, something that has yet to be defined, which will cause this problem. Bulk agents are quite useful for treating constipation. Metamucil (one tablespoon in a glass of water once or twice daily) often gives gentle relief, although it is not palatable to some people. Colace 100 mg by mouth two or three times a day is a stool softener which is particularly helpful if the stools are hard. Bran muffins and other high fiber foods are helpful. Milk of magnesia and other strong laxatives should only be used if simpler regimens of bulk are ineffective. Occasionally, a Fleet enema might need to be taken. If you are prone to this problem on land, take all necessary precautions and bring medication with you on board.

**Vomiting.** Vomiting as a symptom should be separated into several areas. Obviously seasickness will cause vomiting. People usually know if this is what ails them. Early pregnancy may cause morning sickness and vomiting. Has a period been missed? Is there reason to think that this might be the case? Sometimes vomiting is simply an upset stomach from overeating. If so, it will occur only for a short period of time and, once over, the patient will feel better.

A gastroenteritis ("stomach virus") can cause mild vomiting and/or diarrhea. Treat the patient with clear liquids such as water, tea, jello, chicken soup, light toast for a diet, and Lomotil if the diarrhea and cramps are prominent. Avoid milk products, which will only aggravate the illness. If the symptoms don't subside within twenty-four hours, reassess the situation. Patients with this problem do not have severe stomach pain or fever. They aren't feeling too well, but they don't really look sick. Take the patient's temperature to be sure.

Vomiting as an acute illness can be due to food poisoning. This patient is more sick than the patient with a simple upset stomach. Vomiting does not make this patient feel better for long. It usually occurs one to six hours after the ingestion of contaminated food (usually contaminated with bacteria). A fever may be present. The patient will often develop abdominal pain, cramps, and diarrhea along with the vomiting. Maintaining adequate hydration is a high priority here. Most cases are self-limited, that is, they will get better by themselves within a day or two. You should get prompt medical treatment if it doesn't resolve within this time frame or if the patient is unable to retain fluids. A description of the treatment can be found in the section on cramps and diarrhea. See also under Sea Creatures: Ciguatera, Puffer Fish Poisoning, Scombroid Poisoning, and Paralytic Shellfish Poisoning (Red Tide).

Continuous or recurrent vomiting, especially when associated with abdominal pain, can rapidly lead to dehydration and physical collapse. This should be treated as a medical emergency and medical evacuation arranged.

**Seasickness.** Seasickness is the most common affliction aboard boats. Everyone is, therefore, an expert and few know what to do about it. Anyone can become seasick if conditions are bad enough. Those who claim immunity have not likely been caught in a hurricane offshore in a small boat. I have and—although I am usually relatively free from this ailment—I was so sick on that occasion that I prayed for relief. Even death might have been welcomed in lieu of that torture. To grasp a feel for the possibilities, I would like to extract the following from my log of June 1980: "The world seems to have gone mad. We are being thrown about like a rag doll. Now we are rising, rising, lifting to the top of a huge, thirty-five-foot wave. All of a sudden, *Classic* slips over onto her side and we fall. I am in midair, held into my bunk only by the weather cloth as we crash onto our side. The force slams me into the cushion overlying the bunk and the crash sounds as if our fiberglass hull is sure to split in half like an eggshell.

"I am so sick. I've tried Compazine suppositories (five of them), acupressure, pills—nothing works! I wish that I could die. The worst torture thought up by the most infamous tyrant of history could not match this horror. It is like being on a stunt-like amusement park ride, sort of a combination of the whip and ferris wheel; only this ride never ends. No one will let me off. Please, please let me go!

"The wind is screaming a banshee wail like a chorus of a thousand Valkyries gone mad. Then, all of a sudden, it is silent. We are in the eye of the storm. The motion of the boat is still horrible. I must get topsides. I struggle to the companionway, but never make it past the galley sink. I am suddenly so sick and dizzy that I leave my entire soul in that stainless steel basin. Weakly, I crawl back to my bunk."

Needless to say, I survived that episode, a hurricane near Bermuda. Over the years, I have learned new tricks to avoid such an ordeal. The affliction seems to stem from the effect of constant motion on the balancing (vestibular) apparatus in the inner ear. Several factors contribute to its development. Cold, fatigue, fear, other illnesses which weaken the body, and lack of a reference point for the eyes to concentrate on are all influences. Standing on one's feet out in the cockpit helps to stabilize the system. The body unconsciously adapts to each movement of the boat with subtle muscular contractions of the legs diminishing the motion of the head. In addition, if the eyes can concentrate on the horizon they give the brain a reference point. Being placed in charge of the tiller or wheel increases concentration on the task at hand and diminishes the tendency to focus on how you are feeling. Unfortunately, you cannot stay out in the elements forever. Cold and fatigue drive you below. In the cabin, the seasick person is often best tied into his berth. Lee cloths are excellent for this purpose.

The search for a magic potion to make the symptoms of seasickness go away has led to a number of remedies. Some actually work, but often at the cost of side effects that are disabling. Dramamine is an old-fashioned formulation for motion sickness. It works for mild afflictions if taken in advance and every twelve hours during the period of exposure. It often causes sleepiness, however, and it does not work under extreme conditions for most people.

Compazine and Tigan are prescription medications used for nausea in postoperative patients in the hospital. They are available in pill form as well as suppositories and by injection. Again, they aren't so effective if taken after the illness has taken hold. At that time, one cannot take pills and hope to keep them down. Suppositories, although effective for mild to moderate conditions, are not always helpful when the ocean is wild. One Compazine suppository placed in the rectum every six hours (5 mg dosage) may be used.

Scopolamine, sold under the trade name Transderm, is placed as a patch behind the ear and is a popular medication used today. It is often helpful for day trips if taken in advance of the trip, but should not be used for longer periods at sea. When worn over twenty-four hours, continual absorption of the medication increases the incidence of serious side effects such as blurring of vision and mental confusion. It is also totally ineffective for moderately severe conditions such as constantly beating into a heavy sea.

Acupressure, or the application of intense pressure to the palm side of the wrist about three fingerbreadths up from the junction of the wrist and the hand, will often give temporary relief—but only as long as the pressure is held. It is hard to keep it applied for any length of time and, again, it is better for milder conditions than for severe storms. It can, however, be useful in specific short-term circumstances. It can help you get topsides without collapse. The acupressure buttons, which are strapped on with Velcro, have not worked on my crew.

The best medication I have found in my travels is Stugeron. Manufactured by Janssen Pharmaceuticals of Grove, Oxford, England OX12 0DQ as well as in Beerse, Belgium, this antihistamine (cinnarizine 15 mg) is sold throughout Europe for motion sickness. It is not marketed in the United States. Taken as two tablets two hours before sailing and one tablet every eight hours, it is the only medication that has worked for my entire—often seasick— crew. The children's dosage is half the above. I recommend that all long-term sailors use some contact in Europe or Bermuda to find some of this marvelous stuff and get it to you for use as needed. It can be obtained there without a prescription.

**Abdominal Pain.** Abdominal pain can be a frightening symptom. It is almost always, however, easily and medically treatable. If the pain is associated with cramps, the discussion above of cramps and diarrhea applies. Otherwise, the location of the pain and the presence or absence of any tenderness on pressing on the abdomen is the key to diagnosis and treatment. See the specific headings such as heartburn and ulcers, gallbladder infections, appendicitis, diverticulitis, ectopic pregnancy, pelvic infections, and peritonitis for a discussion of how the symptoms differ and which problems are emergency situations.

**Heartburn and Ulcers.** Pain in the upper midabdomen going upward into the lower chest is usually heartburn and can be relieved with an antacid. The patient should take one or two ounces of Maalox or Gelusil. Pain in the left upper part of the abdomen or in the upper midportion of the abdomen is usually pain in the stomach and suggests ulcer-type pain. Sometimes this pain will shoot through into the middle of the back. An antacid should be tried. If it doesn't work within an hour or so, and the pain persists, the patient should see a doctor. Tagamet (an acid blocking medication) is often prescribed by doctors. Zantac may also be used. Such medications offer very effective treatment for ulcers and often eliminate major complications. When ulcer-type symptoms occur, avoid alcohol, aspirin, and Motrin (Advil, etc.). If the condition recurs several times over the next few days, get a medical assessment. Other illnesses in this area can only be diagnosed by sophisticated testing.

**Gallstones and Gallbladder Infections.** Pain in the right upper part of the abdomen can often be due to gallstones. A passing stone is very uncomfortable. Rest, fluids, and light nonfatty meals are helpful, but, if the pain persists for twenty-four hours or more, get the patient to a doctor. If fever occurs as well as tenderness in the right upper portion of the abdomen, then a gallbladder infection may be present. Antibiotics may be needed and are best administered intravenously in a hospital setting. If jaundice occurs (yellow color to the whites of the eyes and later to the skin), either a blocked bile duct (such as can be due to a stone) or a hepatitis may be present. Eat lightly, have plenty of fluids and rest, and get medical assistance as soon as possible. Other illnesses must be carefully ruled out by sophisticated X-ray studies.

**Diverticulitis.** Pain in the left lower part of the abdomen occurs in two age groups. In the over-60 age group this is likely to be diverticulitis, an infection of a weak outpouching (called a diverticulum) in the wall of the large bowel. This can lead to an intra-abdominal abscess. The patient should be seen as soon as possible by a physician, who will probably prescribe antibiotics for mild conditions. A soft diet temporarily until the pain is gone or even just water if the pain is severe will help. Eventually, when things have subsided, plenty of roughage in the diet is helpful. If the pain is severe or persists more than a few hours, see your doctor fast. You may need surgery!

**Ruptured Ovarian Cyst.** In 12- to 18-year-old females, a ruptured ovarian cyst causes lower abdominal pain and usually requires no treatment. If the pain is mild, reassurance and bed rest are all that is needed. Appendicitis (see the section on this ailment) is also common in this age group. Diagnosis should not be delayed if symptoms persist.

**Pelvic Infections.** If the woman is sexually active, has a fever or severe lower abdominal pain (which could be either on the right or left side), then a pelvic infection must be considered and antibiotics will be needed. Seek medical advice. Because of the possibility that an abscess could develop or that an ectopic pregnancy (see below) could be present, do not try to treat this condition without medical assistance and advice.

**Ectopic Pregnancy.** Pain in either the left or the right lower portion of the abdomen, occurring in a woman of childbearing age who has missed a period and/or who has had spotting since the missed period may signal an ectopic pregnancy. This is implantation of the fertilized ovum outside the womb. The fertilized egg is prevented from reaching the uterus and implants (or sets up housekeeping) inside a fallopian tube or the peritoneal (abdominal) cavity. The result is often severe pain or internal bleeding. This may be a surgical emergency and professional help should be obtained as soon as possible.

**Toxemia of Pregnancy.** A pregnant woman in the later stages of pregnancy who develops severe headache, blurring of vision, or midabdominal pain may be developing toxemia of pregnancy (eclampsia). Symptoms may include swelling of the face and arms, although this is not an uncommon development in pregnancy without toxemia. Severe headache, blurred vision, and, most importantly, abdominal pain are the serious warning signs. Doctors still do not know exactly why some women develop toxemia. Some have suggested that it may be due to toxic products produced by the fetus or placenta in response to diminished blood supply. This is because it is often seen as a complication of premature separation of the placenta. Symptoms of its development may, at times, be preceded by vaginal spotting. It can cause kidney failure and swelling of the brain in the mother with edema and convulsions. The development of any of the symptoms mentioned suggests a very serious problem that requires medical evacuation.

**Appendicitis.** Pain in the right lower portion of the abdomen in either sex can mean appendicitis. If the pain has any localized tenderness over it when you press on the right lower portion of the abdomen, then appendicitis must be considered. Often, appendicitis pain begins in the area of the navel and then localizes in the right lower quadrant. It is often associated with fever and a loss of appetite. If the pain persists more than a couple of hours, get a medical examination. This will usually require hospitalization and close observation by trained professionals. Surgery is still the treatment of choice in most cases.

**Peritonitis.** Pain anywhere in the abdomen associated with a tense or rigid abdominal muscle wall and marked tenderness on pushing in may be indicative of peritonitis. This requires surgical attention immediately. Get to a hospital promptly. Medical evacuation will be required if the patient cannot be quickly brought ashore.

**Hernia.** Local pain in the groin, often associated with a bulge or a lump in the groin, may mean the presence of an incarcerated hernia. This means that a weakness is present in the area and a loop of bowel has been pushed through the weakened area. If it is "incarcerated" or imprisoned within the hernia, its blood supply may be compromised and it could die. Have the patient lie down and see if this change of position allows the hernia to reduce. Put an ice pack over the hernia for thirty minutes. If there is little tenderness and no redness over the hernia after the patient has lain down with the ice pack, then gentle pressure on the hernia may help it to reduce. Do not attempt to force this or you may cause damage to the bowel. If the situation does not rapidly resolve with an hour of bed rest, get prompt medical attention.

### BELOW THE WAIST

**Bladder and Kidney Infections.** Pain in the direct area over the pubic bone in the lowest midportion of the abdomen, often in association with frequent urination and/or burning on urination is usually due to a bladder infection. It occurs, most often, in women and girls. Treatment consists of antibiotics. Your doctor may wish to do a urine culture and check to make sure that you have no signs of kidney infection. It may not require immediate medical attention unless the symptoms are very painful. Drinking lots of water and other fluids may help the situation in a matter of hours. A kidney infection is characterized by back pain in the little depression found in the back just below the ribs and off to the side of the backbone (the flank) and is associated with frequent urination and/or burning, with or without fever. This can be more serious and lead to septicemia or a blood infection. Get medical help promptly. Baths and/or swimming may be the source of either bladder or kidney infections in women, and should be avoided for at least a month afterward, if not forever. Bacteria can be washed off the surface of the anus into the bath water and may then colonize the opening of the vagina or urethra. Later growth may allow them to ascend into the bladder. Persons with kidney infections must be seen by a doctor promptly. The possible presence of an un-suspected obstruction to the drainage from the kidney (such as can occur with a kidney stone) combined with the presence of an infection (as indicated by fever and chills) can lead to a life-threatening condition.

**Back Pain.** Back pain made worse by motion such as bending over is due to musculoskeletal pain; this is usually a pulled muscle and will go away with rest. A muscle relaxant such as Flexeril 10 mg three or four times per day is beneficial. A pain reliever such as Advil may also help. If the pain spreads down the back into the buttocks, back of the leg, or lower, it may be due to pressure on one of the spinal nerves. This type of pain is often seen in lumbar disc disease; complete bed rest until the pain has gone is the usual initial treatment. Medical help and advice is needed. Other spinal illnesses might be present. Any sudden loss of sensation in an extremity or loss of function should be considered a medical emergency. Get help fast. Flank pain without fever, unaffected by motion, and often radiating around to the front of the abdomen into the groin, sometimes associated with blood in the urine, may be a kidney stone. It can cause terrible pain which should be treated with pain medication. A medical assessment is advisable.

**Blood in the Urine.** Blood in the urine without pain is a dangerous sign which could indicate cancer; the patient should be evaluated by a urologist. The person should drink plenty of water so the urine doesn't clot up and the bleeding will usually clear. Even if it is a cancer it is nearly always treatable and usually curable, but the patient should get prompt help! Don't assume that because the bleeding has cleared, that it is all better; it needs to be checked! Blood in the urine can also be due to infections and stone disease and, at times prostate obstruction. Diagnosis depends on sophisticated studies.

**Urinary Retention.** Urinary retention (inability to urinate) with an associated discomfort in the lower abdomen is a common problem with older men. It sometimes also occurs in women with urinary infections. A catheter may be needed for relief. Get to your local emergency room for help.

**Testis Pain.** Testicular pain is usually due to an infection (epididymitis). It should be treated with ice or cold packs, rest, and antibiotics. Your urologist or the local emergency room can advise you on the proper medication. Mild testicular pain in young men is often due to congestion from overexcitement in the previous eight to twelve hours. It will pass on its own.

In children and young adults, a twisted testicle may occur (torsion). Pain in the testicle in this age group requires immediate evaluation. Its hallmark is that the pain occurs suddenly and on examination the affected testis is found to be, at times, higher than its mate. It can be gently untwisted if you try first one way then the other. Otherwise, simply put on cold packs until you can get to the hospital. Treatment must be instituted by a urologist within six hours to save the testicle. Prompt medical help must be sought, and sophisticated tests may be needed to clarify the diagnosis.

Any firm lump or mass in the testicle should be examined by a urologist promptly. Many are simply hydroceles (fluid filled sacs). Light from a flashlight can be seen through the mass defining its character. This does not require emergency treatment. Cancer of the testicle, however, is a rapidly fatal condition which can be *cured* by early detection and treatment. Don't hide from this possibility and wait to see if it goes away. Lumps do not go away!

**Vaginal Bleeding.** Vaginal bleeding is associated with miscarriages in young adult women and with tumors in older women. Simply an irregular period must also be considered. Mild bleeding can be checked when you reach shore. More serious bleeding requires immediate bed rest and a call should be made on the emergency radio network for a medevac. Saturation of a pad or more per hour must be considered serious bleeding. Any vaginal bleeding during pregnancy should be considered a medical emergency until proved otherwise.

**Vaginitis.** Vaginitis or itching and burning in the vagina is usually associated with an infection caused by a fungal organism called monilia. It can result from treatment with an antibiotic for any illness or as a result of environmental factors. Antifungal medications such as Monistat vaginal tablets are often recommended. Other causes of vaginitis

occur, but require an examination by a doctor for diagnosis. Although these conditions cause discomfort, they
are not emergency situations.

**Blood in the Stool.** Blood in the stool (mixed up in the stool)
can mean bleeding in the bowel. At times, it is red or
reddish-brown and is clearly blood. At other times, it is
black in color indicating that  the bleeding occurred high
up in the stomach. Iron-containing pills will also cause
black stools. Possible causes of bleeding include inflam-
matory bowel disease in younger people, infections, diver-
ticulosis, ischemic bowel disease, colonic ulcers, or a
cancer. The person having this sympton should be checked
as soon as you can get to a hospital. Blood on the toilet
paper or on the outside of a brown stool is usually caused
by an irritation or hemorrhoid and is of no immediate
concern. The person should still see a doctor for a rectal
examination within a reasonable period of time.

**Anal Irritations.** Anal irritations can be very effectively
treated with 0.5% hydrocortisone cream applied two or
three times daily until the discomfort has gone. Zinc oxide
cream is also very effective and acts as a seal to prevent
rectal contents from irritating the sensitive skin around
the anus.

**Hemorrhoids.** Hemorrhoids (thrombosed veins in the anal
area) can be treated with warm soaks in a large pan or tub.
In this area, pilonidal cysts (formed near the coccyx or
tailbone) and anal fissures can become infected. The principles are the same—soak, soak, soak!

**Gout.** The great toe is the final localized anatomic site
which we will look at. In older people, especially men, a

painful swelling of the great toe, often accompanied by redness, may be due to gout. Caused by a high level of a by-product of protein metabolism called uric acid (which collects in and irritates the joints), this can be a disabling illness which may be quickly alleviated. Most cases of gout can be treated temporarily with rest, ice, and elevation. Tylenol or Advil may be tried, but medical advice should be sought as far more effective prescription medications are available.

## SUNBURN AND HEATSTROKE

**Sunburn.** The major cause of disability in the sunny isles of the Caribbean is sunburn. People go south for the winter with one thought in mind: to soak up as much sun as possible. The idea seems to linger that the more tan you get, the longer it will last. Unfortunately, this idea can ruin an otherwise wonderful vacation. The tropical sun is much stronger than most people from temperate climates are accustomed to. Everyone except brown- or black-skinned peoples should apply a #20 sun block for the first day or two. A #15 sun block should be used for the next two or three days, and a #8 sunscreen for the next two or three days. A person will tan using such a regimen and may do so without the risk of a severe burn. Zinc oxide works well to protect lips, nose, and other sensitive areas. Once a good protective tan has started, then a less strong sun protection may or may not be needed depending on the fairness of the person's skin. Lotions containing aloe are usually soothing to the burn. It should be noted, however, that one can even burn through a white T-shirt. Good protective clothing should be worn by the fair-skinned individual.

Cancer of the skin has recently come into prominence. Skin cancers are occurring with increased frequency and are a public health concern. The reason for the increase appears to be that more people have the leisure time to spend increasing amounts of time in the sun. In addition, people are living longer, and it is more common for the elderly to get cancer. There is also some evidence that the ozone in the upper levels of the atmosphere is being destroyed by chemical compounds found in pressurized aerosol cans, refrigerators, and air conditioners. These otherwise harmless gases apparently are collecting at upper levels of the atmosphere and combining chemically with the ozone. The ozone has, in the past, acted to block the more harmful ultraviolet rays of the sun from reaching earth. Diminished concentrations of ozone mean that the sun can cause more harm than it has in the past. Your crew should be encouraged to wear sun screen!

**Heatstroke.** Heatstroke is a collapse of body systems due to prolonged exposure to heat and fluid loss. The subject becomes weak and feels faint. He may lose consciousness, vomit, or even have a convulsion. The best treatment is prevention. Making every effort to keep cool by providing shade and/or a breeze, as well as avoiding undue exercise in the sun or in an overheated environment will help prevent this potentially devastating illness. Drinking plenty of fluids is helpful. Orange juice and fruit juices, which contain some electrolytes and natural sugars, can be helpful. Water is most important. The reaction of the body to heatstroke involves a number of sophisticated reactions. The most important is a loss of fluids due to increased sweating without adequate replacement. This causes an increase in sodium and other electrolytes in the body. Even though sodium is lost through sweat, more water than salt is lost. Blood volume falls and there is an increase in the concentration of toxins in the body as there is less fluid for the kidneys to use to eliminate waste. This combination of events disturbs basic cellular reactions. In addition, a buildup of internal body heat occurs which can damage the heat-sensitive enzymes needed for the body to function. It used to be taught that salt should be taken to prevent heatstroke. This is because there is some salt loss from perspiration. Current thinking is that this should *not* be done. The net loss is water, not salt. By adding salt to the diet or by taking salt tablets, you increase your body's need for water and you increase the sodium imbalance in the body. Gatoraid used to be recommended, since it contains many of the electrolytes lost. Again, it has been found that simply drinking water is the most helpful. Keep in the shade, rinse yourself with cooling seawater, and drink plenty of fluids. The first reaction of heatstroke is a failure in the system to regulate temperature and blood pressure. The blood pools in the small vessels all over the body, the pressure goes down, and the person loses consciousness. In its most extreme, the body will lose liver and kidney function, the person will go into a coma, and he will not recover. In the case of collapse get the person to a hospital promptly. Treatment is often difficult and requires hospitalization, intravenous fluids, and careful management.

## POISONINGS AND DANGEROUS CRITTERS

A number of oceanic creatures have defense systems that can incapacitate and injure a human being. Brief notes on each with recommended treatments for their contact follows.* Much of the material presented here is based on a

---

* Significant material on fish poisonings was sent to the author by Dr. Y. Hokama, Professor, Department of Pathology, University of Hawaii School of Medicine. Of great value to the serious student is an article written by Dr. Hokama in the *Journal of Clinical Laboratory Analysis* published in February 1988 (2:44-50).

number of texts and articles on the subject, including the excellent *Medical Toxicology: Diagnosis and Treatment of Human Poisoning*, by Matthew J. Ellenhorn and Donald G. Barceloux.

**Jellyfish.** Jellyfish have stinging cells on the end of their tentacles. If stung, wash with seawater, remove the tentacles with forceps or pliers, apply alcohol to the nematocysts (stingers) stuck to the skin, then apply dry baking soda, flour, talcum powder, or shaving cream and scrape the nematocysts off with a sharp knife. Do not use your fingers for this. Wash with fresh water (only after all the nematocysts are off). Pain may respond to hot water soaks for thirty minutes. You may apply cortisone cream for residual local skin irritation. The patient should see a doctor if signs of infection occur over the next twenty-four to forty-eight hours.

Portuguese man-of-war injuries are among the most dangerous of jellyfish stings and may occur in Atlantic or Pacific waters. They cause intense local pain with blisters occurring at the site of injury. Weakness, vomiting, muscle spasms, and pain in the back and abdomen can occur. On occasion, depression of the heart and difficulty with breathing can occur. Children are affected most severely. Vinegar is effective in paralyzing the nematocysts and allowing their removal; it may be used instead of alcohol. Hospitalization may be required for this type of injury.

**Coral.** Coral, especially fire coral, can cause severe burning upon contact. Wash with seawater, apply alcohol, then apply hydrogen peroxide, and finally cortisone cream (0.5% hydrocortisone). Antibiotics are probably not necessary. Severe lacerations may, however, require surgical exploration with removal of the fragments of coral.

**Sea Urchins.** Sea urchins and stinging cones will penetrate the skin with their spines. They cause intense pain, redness, and swelling. Remove all spines, apply vinegar soaks, then soak in hot, fresh water like a puncture wound and see a doctor for antibiotics if the punctures are severe.

**Other Stinging Fish.** Scorpion fish, stingrays, and catfish can inject a poison. Most injuries occur when fishermen try to take them off a hook. They cause local pain, swelling, and pain up the arm. Muscle cramps, weakness, and tremor may occur. Stone fish can cause fatalities through respiratory failure. Stingrays also can cause severe systemic symptoms. Wash the wound with seawater and encourage it to bleed. Clean out any foreign matter. Soak in very hot fresh water (without blistering the skin) for thirty to sixty minutes. The toxin is destroyed by heat. Antibiotics may be needed if signs of infection occur. Stone fish stings require antivenom. This may be obtained from the Steinhart Aquarium in San Francisco (415-221-8014) or Sea World in San Diego (619-222-0411).

**Sea Snakes.** Sea snakes are very poisonous. Their bite leaves tiny punctures that do not hurt initially. Sea snakes are related to the cobra on land. Difficulty in breathing and paralysis follows a sea snake bite within thirty to sixty minutes. Treatment is urgent. Lower the extremity, quickly put on a tourniquet to block venous return, and give antivenom promptly (available from the Department of Health, Commonwealth Serum Lab in Melbourne, Australia). Get the patient evacuated to a hospital.

**Ciguatera.** A localized form of food poisoning, ciguatera is associated with eating fish in tropical waters. The organism that causes it is distributed as far north as Bermuda and as far south as Buenos Aires (35° north to 35° south). In some areas, reef fish, which feed off coral, ingest a highly fatal toxin produced by a tiny organism (called a dinoflagellate) attached to algae. It causes half of all food poisoning related to fish in the United States. This toxin, which doesn't seem to bother the fish in the slightest, may, on occasion, be death to man. It becomes even more strongly concentrated in the carnivorous fish such as barracuda, grouper, snapper, jacks, and amberjacks, since they eat contaminated reef fish. The toxin is not inactivated by cooking the fish.

Symptoms may occur anywhere from ten minutes to twelve hours after eating the contaminated fish. Nausea, vomiting, abdominal pain, and diarrhea may be followed by numbness and tingling of the hands and feet, weakness, and dizziness. Blurred vision, increased salivation, and unsteadiness on one's feet occur. The numbness and pins and needles sensation noted above is considered the hallmark of ciguatera poisoning and differentiates it from other forms of food poisoning. Hypotension and slowing of the heart with difficulty in breathing may occur. This may later be followed by high blood pressure and rapid heart action. Increased sensitivity to cold may occur as a later phenomenon. The treatment is to induce vomiting and give fluids. Professional help may be of assistance. Medical evacuation should be arranged.

Many people recommend eating small fish (less than five pounds), since the larger fish have higher concentrations of the toxin. Others suggest that you ask locals if it is okay to eat the local reef fish. Since it is such a serious problem, and since the locals are often the ones who get sick, I would recommend that you not eat any reef fish or predatory fish such as barracuda, grouper, amberjack, jacks, snapper, or moray eel in tropical waters! Milder symptoms have even been shown after eating the browsing fish such as surgeonfish. I suggest that you concentrate on catching pelagic or deepwater fish such as dolphin (not the mammal) between island stops and leave the reef fish to the locals. Treatment should be symptomatic and professional help should be obtained. More serious illnesses occur with high concentrations of the toxin, and the eating of fish livers, roe, or entrails causes more fatalities. Otherwise, fatalities are uncommon, but persistence of the symptoms and weakness may occur for weeks.

Dr. Y. Hokama of the University of Hawaii has reported the development of an enzyme assay for the detection of ciguatoxin in contaminated fish that has shown great promise. Currently, the test is only applicable to large fish processing plants, but Dr. Hokama is beginning trials of a new one-step test which can be used by individual fishermen. He hopes to have it available in the early 1990s.

**Scombroid Poisoning.** Inadequately refrigerated fish may cause a form of poisoning called scombroid. Bacteria in the fish convert a normally present amino acid (histidine) to histamine causing acute flushing of the skin, itching, headache, and dizziness. Vomiting and diarrhea may occur. Generalized itching and hives may be prominent. Occasionally, difficulty in breathing may occur. Fish such as tuna, mackerel, bonito, skipjack, and mahimahi are associated with this illness. If symptoms occur shortly after eating fish, get the patient to vomit. Get medical help; cimetidine (Tagamet) is often effective and may be given at the hospital.

**Puffer Fish Poisoning.** Puffer fish are highly toxic and should not be eaten. Fugu, or Japanese puffer fish, is a delicacy in Japan. It requires special preparation by experts, but, even so, numerous poisonings have been reported. It is often served raw in sashimi. Japanese restaurants on both coasts of the United States and in Hawaii sometimes serve it as a specialty. Pins-and-needles sensations, numbness, sweating, chest pain, and paralysis can occur after about an hour. Induce vomiting early, give laxatives and enemas. Don't eat this stuff!

**Paralytic Shellfish Poisoning (Red Tide).** Another form of food poisoning is found on both the northeast coast of the United States and on the West Coast up into Alaska. This is red tide or paralytic shellfish poisoning. Mussels, clams, and the stomachs of scallops (not usually the part eaten) may contain a highly toxic poison that paralyzes the muscles and can prevent breathing. Symptoms usually start with numbness and tingling around the mouth and in the hands or feet. Vomiting and abdominal pain may follow; numbness in the fingers followed by difficulty in movements and breathing then occur. State health departments often test for such problems by injecting ground up clams into mice. Wide areas of coast may thus be closed to shellfishing. If an area is closed, do not eat the shellfish. (Lobster and crabs are not involved in this problem.) Immediate transportation to a hospital is vital so that the ill patient can be put on a respirator.

Clams and mussels can also be a source of hepatitis. The wise sailor or boatsman will eat his clams from commercial purveyors who are usually aware of the problem areas and stay away from them. If you must gather clams or mussels on your own, I would strongly advise checking with the VHF weather channel which lists shellfish closing in your area. Offshore islands are often where the red tide blooms start so that these are not given any magic protection simply because they are remote. They are harder to reach and sample by the marine scientists involved and the shellfish may not have been checked. The summer months are the worst offenders, but there are places where red tide is present year-round. At least check carefully with the locals. Hopefully, a word to the wise here will be sufficient.

A number of different toxins have been reported associated with PSP poisoning. Work is currently in progress to try to develop an enzyme assay method of detecting these toxins. Eventually, these may be available for simplified testing in the field.

**Insect Bites.** The bites of mosquitoes, no-see-ums, black flies, and other insects cause tiny, painful, itchy sores. Prevention is preferred using insect repellent, screens, and long sleeves, but if you have been badly bitten, take an antihistamine such as Actifed or Benadryl. One dose will usually eliminate the itching of the local reaction within an hour. Dale Nouse, an editor of *Practical Sailor*, relates that Vitamin B1 (thiamine), taken daily, discourages the little critters from biting. I have had no personal experience with this.

Bees, wasps, hornets, and yellow jackets inject a powerful toxin. The amount is, fortunately, small unless one is stung by a large number of insects. Local reaction varies in intensity. Beestings can be treated by pulling out the stinger with smooth forceps (if you can see it), putting ice on the local injury, and, if you are getting a lot of swelling, taking an antihistamine. Severe allergic reactions can cause death. If you start to have some trouble breathing, get to a hospital. Early treatment with prednisone or epinephrine may be needed. People who are known to have asthma should be tested and desensitized to beestings.

Such people should obtain an epinephrine aerosol spray and sublingual isoproterenol tablets from a physician and carry them for emergency use.

**Scorpion Stings.** Scorpions have a long, segmented tail with a stinger at the tip. They climb rather than burrow and prefer areas around trees. Scorpions are predominantly found in the Southwest, but may also be seen in Florida and, in the East, as far north as Virginia. The symptom of scorpion stings is local pain lasting about ten hours. Children are more seriously affected and many become overexcited and develop convulsions. Information about an antivenom developed from goats is available from the Antivenom Production Laboratory, Department of Botany and Microbiology, Arizona State University (602-965-1457 or 6443). As mentioned in chapter 1, I had the experience of treating a presumed scorpion sting with hot soaks. Scorpion stings may be treated by putting the affected extremity in hot water (as hot as you can stand it). The toxin may be heat sensitive and, if so, the pain and swelling will subside. This is anecdotal and cannot be considered conclusive information. Otherwise treat like a beesting.

**Spider Bites.** The black widow spider, small with a round, shiny, black body, has a red hourglass mark on back of its round, globular body. Its bite causes slight redness and swelling locally. Within ten minutes, cramps and severe pain spread from the bite site to areas adjacent and then to the rest of the body. Anxiety, headache, nausea, tightness of the chest, and difficulty with breathing may occur. Children and the elderly have the most severe reactions. It can, occasionally, be fatal. An antivenom is available. Tetanus immunization should be updated at the time of the bite.

**Snake Bites.** The coral snake may be found in remote shoreline areas in most southern states. It has red, yellow, and black stripes encircling its body. The coral snake bite causes little local reaction. Several hours after the bite, lightheadedness or drowsiness followed by tremor, weakness, and nausea occur. This may progress to paralysis of breathing or convulsions. Get medical evacuation promptly. Capture the snake for identification, if you can do so safely. Pressure wrapping and immobilization of the extremity have been reported to slow the spread of the toxin.

**Animal Bites.** Animal bites by dogs, cats, and wild animals should be cleansed and soaked in very warm to hot water (without burning the injured part) for at least thirty to forty-five minutes. Antibiotic treatment should be considered if the wound is more than just a scratch. Human bites are especially dangerous and require antibiotics. If the animal cannot be carefully observed for ten days after the bite, and if it is known to be a species that can carry rabies (dogs, cats, foxes, squirrels, raccoons, and bats), then rabies vaccination and tetanus immunization should be initiated.

**Leeches.** Leeches are freshwater annoyances associated with muddy bottoms. They latch onto the body and proceed to invade the skin to feed on blood. They can be easily removed by sprinkling salt on them. They will quickly curl up and can then be brushed off.

# 4. How to Handle Life-Threatening Problems

## CPR (CARDIOPULMONARY RESUSCITATION)

I believe that it is of great importance to take your health and that of your crew seriously. It is not within the scope of this book to teach cardiopulmonary resuscitation (CPR); you should learn it before you leave home in one of the many CPR courses run by hospitals, the American Heart Association, the Red Cross, and other volunteer organizations. At least two members of a boat's crew should have this information.

A quick review follows. Basic life support involves establishing an airway, providing artificial respiration, and promoting circulation of the blood in the absence of effective heart action. If the victim is unconscious, check to see if he is breathing. Look for a rise and fall in his chest; listen for breathing by placing your ear close to his mouth; feel for air coming from his mouth with your cheek. If the person is not breathing, lay him flat on his back on a firm surface, tilt his head backward to open the airway (see figure 4). If the person then breathes spontaneously, just keep the airway open. If not, pinch the victim's nostrils with your finger and thumb, cover his mouth (which has been pulled open) with your mouth and blow out forcefully four times into the victim to expand his lungs (figure 5). Feel for a pulse in the neck (carotid; see figure 6). If a pulse

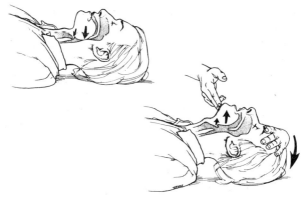

*Fig. 4. Opening the airway:* top, *airway obstruction produced by the tongue and epiglottis;* bottom, *relief by head-tilt/chin-lift. From* Healthcare Provider's Manual for Basic Life Support, © *American Heart Association. Reproduced with permission.*

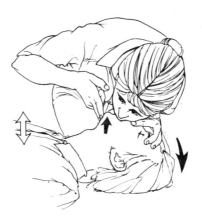

*Fig. 5. Mouth-to-mouth rescue breathing. From* Healthcare Provider's Manual for Basic Life Support, © *American Heart Association. Reproduced with permission.*

is present, continue breathing for the victim and recheck his pulse every minute. If no pulse is felt, then start chest compression. Find the midsternum (breastbone) by placing your middle and index fingers in the notch at the base of the chest where the ribs come together (see figure 7). Place the heel of your other hand beside your fingers above the notch (see figure 8). You should then compress the midsternum with the heel of your left hand, with your arm held rigidly straight directly over the patient, and your right hand on top of your left. (figures 9-10) The weight of your upper body provides the compression and pushes the breastbone in about one and one-half to two inches (see figure 11). Releasing the pressure allows blood to return to the heart. Repeat eighty to one hundred times per minute. Breathe twice for the victim every fifteen compressions (if you are alone) and once every five compressions if two people are attempting to revive the person (see figures 12-13). *Practice on specially constructed dummies in a CPR program is vital. Do not practice on healthy individuals; serious injury can occur.*

**Drowning.** Drowning victims should be cared for in the same manner as other unconscious persons. Turn the victim on his back and initiate CPR as above. Because it is often difficult to determine how long a victim has been apneic (unable to breathe), one should always attempt CPR in a drowning victim unless there is strong evidence of prolonged death such as surface decomposition. The victims are often young and healthy. Cold water and the diving reflex slow a person's heart rate and constrict the blood vessels leading to the surface areas of the body. This diverts blood from the skin, limbs, and intestines to the more critical centers such as the heart and brain. These reflexes permit the body to survive longer than would

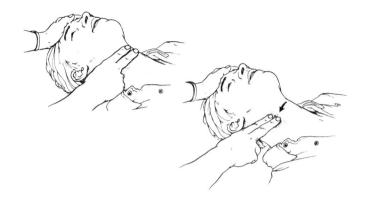

*Fig. 6. Locating the carotid pulse. From* Healthcare Provider's Manual for Basic Life Support, © *American Heart Association. Reproduced with permission.*

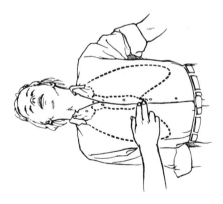

*Fig. 7. External chest compressions: locating the notch where the rib margin meets the sternum. From* Healthcare Provider's Manual for Basic Life Support, © *American Heart Association. Reproduced with permission.*

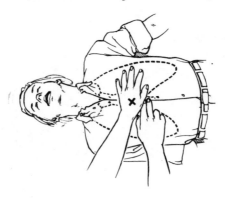

*Fig. 8. External chest compressions: locating the correct hand position on the lower half of the sternum. From* Health-care Provider's Manual for Basic Life Support, © *American Heart Association. Reproduced with permission.*

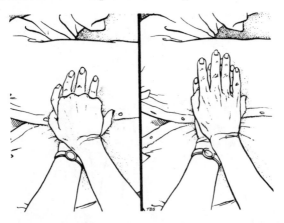

*Fig. 9. Hand positions for external chest compressions. From* Healthcare Provider's Manual for Basic Life Support, © *American Heart Association. Reproduced with permission.*

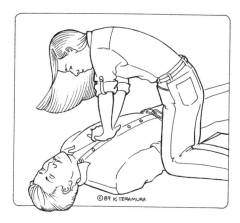

Fig. 10. *Proper position of rescuer: shoulders directly over victim's sternum; elbows locked.*

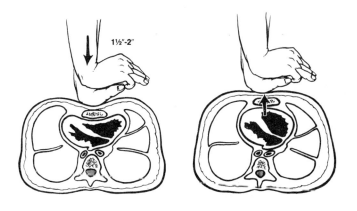

Fig. 11. *External chest compressions: sternum compressed to a depth of 1 1/2 - 2 inches.* From Healthcare Provider's Manual for Basic Life Support, © *American Heart Association. Reproduced with permission.*

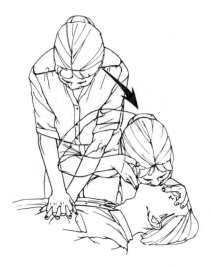

*Fig. 12. One-rescuer adult CPR: fifteen compressions are alternated with two ventilations. From* Healthcare Provider's Manual for Basic Life Support, © *American Heart Association. Reproduced with permission.*

otherwise be expected. Numerous reports of survival with full neurologic recovery after prolonged periods of apnea under such circumstances have been published.

**Electric Shock.** Electric shock may lead to cardiac arrest. Clear the victim from the source of electricity carefully without endangering yourself. You may use a nonconductive object like a wooden stick for this purpose. Then carefully determine if the victim is unconscious and/or breathing. Check for a pulse and institute CPR as needed. Lightning acts as a massive direct current countershock to the heart and causes depolarization of the heart muscle. The heart may resume beating spontaneously afterward and may well

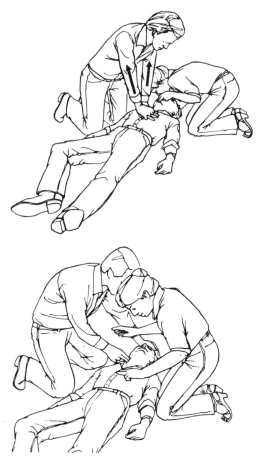

*Fig. 13. Two-rescuer CPR:* above, *pause after the fifth external chest compression;* below, *compressor and ventilator switch positions. From* Healthcare Provider's Manual for Basic Life Support, © *American Heart Association. Reproduced with permission.*

respond to prompt CPR. Victims who do not have cardiac arrest have a good chance for recovery.

**Airway Obstruction and Choking on Food.** Partially chewed food can obstruct the breathing passage. The victim may be unable to speak, breathe, or cough. If he can still get air and is coughing, leave him alone. Watch him and unless serious distress is indicated by a weak, ineffective cough, high-pitched noises when breathing in, and increased breathing difficulties, don't interfere. If increased difficulty with breathing is obvious, then use the Heimlich maneuver. Stand behind the victim, put your arms around his waist, and make a fist with one hand. With the thumb against the victim's abdomen (in the middle above the navel), grab the fist with the other hand and pull quickly and hard. Use an upward pull (see figure 14). Repeat the thrust until the foreign body is pushed out or the victim loses consciousness. If the victim is unconscious, lay him on his back, straddle his thighs, place the heel of one hand against his abdomen (again midline above the navel), and place the other hand over the first. Press into the abdomen with a quick upward thrust (see figure 15). Six to ten thrusts may be needed to clear the airway.

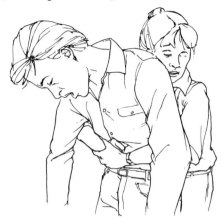

*Fig. 14. Heimlich maneuver administered to a conscious victim. From* Healthcare Provider's Manual for Basic Life Support, © *American Heart Association. Reproduced with permission.*

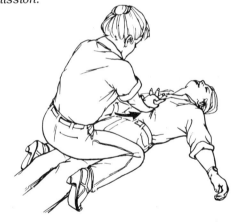

*Fig. 15. Heimlich maneuver administered to an unconscious victim. From* Healthcare Provider's Manual for Basic Life Support, © *American Heart Association. Reproduced with permission.*

# 5. Medications and Supplies

## SIDE EFFECTS FROM MEDICATIONS

Allergy to any of a number of medications can occur. This can take several forms. The most common is a skin rash or hives. This may be a pink, bumpy rash over the upper part of the body on the trunk or on the extremities. Itching may or may not be present. A fever, which was not there before the treatment, may be another form of presentation. Occasionally, jaundice may be seen (yellow color to the eyes and/or skin). If any of the above do occur, stop the particular medication and stay off all medications until the symptoms begin to resolve. Treatment of itching or hives with Benadryl 50 mg by mouth three times a day is appropriate. Serious allergic reactions require medical help.

At times, other side effects of medications can occur. Diarrhea sometimes is an offshoot of ampicillin treatment. If the primary illness is mild, stop the antibiotic. If the primary illness is major, keep up the antibiotic despite the diarrhea and treat the diarrhea with Lomotil. Antibiotics also cause vaginitis in some women. Simply continue the antibiotic and see your doctor for Monistat to treat the vaginitis concomitantly. More severe side effects to medications can include wheezing, difficulty in breathing (treat as under asthma) or complete circulatory collapse. Muscle aches and joint pains with or without fever, or jaundice may occur. Bleeding from the stomach (patient vomits blood or has black stools), and aplastic anemia (destruction of the ability of the body to produce red and white blood cells) are of even greater concern. Obviously, these side effects are extremely serious and the offending medication should be stopped. Immediate medical attention must be sought.

Finally, as mentioned in the Preface, pregnant women and nursing mothers should never take any medication without discussing it with their obstetrician. A medication that is normally safe and reliable may cause birth defects in early pregnancy. The medication may be transmitted to the fetus or the nursing baby who may not be able to tolerate it because of the stage of development.

## MEDICATIONS AND SUPPLIES

A complete medical kit is of great value. The following story illustrates how carrying such a kit aboard helped us save a family vacation.

I waited anxiously in the heat at the airport in Antigua. It had been five weeks since I had seen my family. The ocean crossing had taken its toll, but now was to be a time of pure pleasure. This was my first visit to the Caribbean and it would be so for the family as well. As they climbed the ramp leading to the terminal, I could see a strain on my wife Cindy's face. John's face was pale and he was walking slowly holding his abdomen. We checked them through customs and I was told that our eleven-year-old had begun to have abdominal pain on the plane ride down. With concerns about possible appendicitis or other intra-abdominal emergencies, I immediately thought of making arrangements to fly us all back to Boston for his surgery.

"Slow down," I said to myself. "At least you've been through this before." We drove past the local hospital in St. John and I knew that I could never bring him into that ramshackle collection of sheds. When we got aboard *Free Spirit*, I carefully examined him. Where did it hurt? He pointed to the upper midabdomen. Was it tender when I pushed on it? Yes. Did it hurt when I pushed in the lower abdomen on either side? No. When I pushed in down there and let it go? No. Well, at least he had no evidence of peritonitis. Upper midabdominal pain was suggestive that he had an ulcer and the tenderness indicated that it might be eroding into or through the wall of the stomach or duodenum (upper small bowel). Fortunately, I had a rather complete medical kit aboard. Immediately, we started him on antacids and Tagamet by mouth. This medication acts by blocking the production of stomach acid. Without acid, the ulcer could heal. Within twenty-four hours, the pain was gone. We kept him on a bland diet for two weeks and kept up the Tagamet for the same time and then tapered it off completely. He has never had a problem since. Without that medication aboard and the knowledge of when to use it, our vacation would undoubtedly have been cut short. Furthermore, if he wasn't started on the medication promptly, he might have perforated the ulcer and created the need for open surgery.

## THE BOATER'S MEDICAL KIT

A *P* after a medication in the list below indicates the need for a prescription to obtain it. Ask your pharmacist to label each medication with the name of the product, its usual dosage, and a date of expiration (not the date of purchase which is often used). Antibiotics rapidly lose their effectiveness after expiration and, although products which are outdated by a month may still be effective, I would not recommend the use of a product which is a year out of date. Conditions of storage must also be considered. I would not recommend that many biologically active products such as antibiotics be exposed to extreme temperatures such as those which can be reached in a closed boat cabin in the hot sun. Either keep them in a plastic sealed container in your icebox or refrigerator, or find a cool place in the bilge for them.

70% alcohol
alcohol swabs
elastic bandage (2")
Betadine (pharmadine) swabs
butterfly bandages
adhesive bandages
cotton balls
eye patches
gauze pads 4" × 4"—sterile
gauze roller bandage (2")
oral thermometer
tape (2" nylon)
petroleum jelly gauze (3" wide strips)

Actifed (Allerest is a substitute.)
aloe sunburn cream or lotion
ampicillin 500 mg *P*
antacids: Gelusil tablets or Maalox
aspirin (for headaches)
Benadryl 25 mg (Allerest tablets contain an antihistamine and decongestant and may be a substitute.)
Compazine suppositories 5 mg *P* (Dramamine is a substitute.)
codeine sulfate 30 mg *P* (Percogesic may be used for mild to moderate headache or pain.)
Colace 100 mg *P*
chewable vitamin C 500 mg

dicloxacillin 250 mg *P* (Allergic reactions are common
    since this is a penicillin.)

erythromycin 500 mg *P*

Flexeril 10 mg *P*

hydrogen peroxide, one bottle

0.5% hydrocortisone cream (No prescription is needed.)

Imodium (for diarrhea)

Keflex 500 mg *P*

Metamucil

Monistat vaginal tablets *P*

Motrin 400 mg (useful for premenstrual cramps) *P*
    (Advil is a nonprescription substitute for Motrin.)

Neosporin eye ointment *P*

Neosporin, polymyxin B, hydrocortisone eardrops *P*

Phenergan expectorant with codeine *P* (Robitussin
    DM is a reasonable substitute.)

prednisone 10 mg *P*

Stugeron (cinnarizine 15 mg)—available only in Europe
    (Dramamine is a locally available substitute.)

sunburn lotions (#8, #15, and #20 sunburn protection)
    Get PABA-free lotion if anyone is allergic to the
    PABA.

Slo-Phyllin 250 mg *P* (Primatene tablets are weak, but
    effective substitutes; also, Bronkaid Mist, which
    contains epinephrine, is helpful for asthmatics.)

1% silver sulfadiazine cream *P*

tetracycline 250 mg *P*

Tagamet 300 mg *P*

Tylenol, Extra-Strength

vinegar

zinc oxide cream

I would encourage you to ask for the product literature on
each of the above medications. Save the literature and

familiarize yourself with the adverse reactions or side effects listed. This will protect you from reactions not listed here.

Going to sea has always had risk, but then again, so do most worthwhile things in life. With the technology and knowledge available today, the boater can markedly diminish those risks. It is my sincere hope that this little book will assist that process.

# Index